FOUNTAINS OF YOUTH

HOW TO LIVE LONGER & HEALTHIER

FOUNTAINS OF YOUTH

HOW TO LIVE LONGER & HEALTHIER

BY THE EDITORS OF RONIN PUBLISHING

RONIN PUBLISHING, INC. BOX 1035, BERKELEY, CA 94701

FOUNTAINS OF YOUTH: How to Live Longer & Healthier
ISBN: 0-914171-76-3
Copyright © 1996 by Ronin Publishing, Inc.

Ronin Publishing, Inc.
Post Office Box 1035
Berkeley, California 94701

Project Editors:	Sebastian Orfali and Beverly Potter
Manuscript Editors:	Mary Lou Sumberg and Ginger Ashworth
Technical Editors:	Chadd Everone, Ph.D., Ward Dean, M.D., and John A. Mann
Charts, Illustrations:	B.C. Capps
Cover Design:	Brian Groppe
Page Composition:	Candy Avila, Erik Linden
Draft Manuscript:	Chadd Everone, Ph.D.

Printed in the United States of America by Delta Litho
First printing 1996

9 8 7 6 5 4 3 2 1

PERMISSION NOTICES

Cristofalo, V., et al., "Molecular Biology of Aging," *Surgical Clinics of North America*, vol. 74:1, pp. 1-21, Feb. 1994.

Dean, W., *Biological Aging Measurement: Clinical Applications*, Center for Bio-Gerontology, 1992. Fig: 8.1.

Everone, C.A., *Life-Extension and Control of Aging Program: Manual of Principles and Procedures*, Foundation for Infinite Survival, 1981. Figs: 1.1, 1.2, 1.3, 1.4, 1.5, 2.3, 3.1, 3.3, 5.3, 8.2, 8.3, 8.4, 8.5, 8.6, 8.7, 8.8, 9.1, 10.1.

Gascoigne, B. and Irwin, J., *Smart Ways to Stay Young and Healthy*, Ronin Publishing, 1992.

Gruman, Gerald J. "A History of Ideas about the Prolongation of Life: Evolution of Prolongevity Hypotheses to 1800," *Transactions of the American Philosophical Society*, vol. 56:9, pp. 1-102, 1966.

Karuna Corporation Technical Sheet, "Free Radicals and Antioxidant Coping Mechanisms," *Professional Information Series,* 1986.

Mann, J., *Secrets of Life Extension: How to Halt or Reverse the Aging Process and Live a Long and Healthy Life*, And/Or Press and Harbor Publishing, 1980. Figs: 1.8, 2.2, 2.5, 4.1, 5.2, 6.1, 6.2, 7.1, 7.2, 7.3.

Null, G. and Feldman, M., *Reverse the Aging Process Naturally*, Villard Books, 1993.

Pelton, R., *Mind Foods and Smart Pills*, Doubleday, 1989. Fig: 4.4.

Rockstein, Morris, et al, "Comparative Biology and Evolution of Aging," *Handbook of the Biology of Aging* (1st ed., Finch, C.E. and Hayflick, L., eds.), pp. 9, Van Nostrand Reinhold, 1977. Fig: 2.4.

Walford, R.L. and Walford, L., *The Anti-Aging Plan: Strategies and Recipes for Extending Your Healthy Years*, Four Walls Eight Windows, 1994. Fig: 3.2.

Wolfe, S.L., *Introduction to Cell Biology*, Wadsworth Publishing, 1983. Figs: 1.7, 4.2, 4.3, 5.1.

INTRODUCTION

BY WARD DEAN, M.D.

The modern "life-extension" movement took off like a rocket in 1982, with the publication and publicity campaign surrounding Durk Pearson and Sandy Shaw's smash best-seller, *Life Extension–A practical Scientific Approach.* What is not well-known to many in the life extension community is that two years prior to the release of the Pearson-Shaw book, a little-known book by John Mann titled *Secrets of Life Extension* (SOL) was published. With regard to content, SOL was as much a landmark book as was *Life Extension,* and in many areas was even superior to the Pearson-Shaw book.

Secrets of Life Extension was regarded by many as the most comprehensive and clearly-written life-extension book that had ever been published at that time. It included thorough discussions of nutrition, antioxidants, free radical control, preventing immune system decline and mental senility, combating "death hormone" (DECO) with natural agents, and undoing cross-linkage in DNA and connective tissues. Straight-forward appraisals of anti-aging therapies such as hormone replacement, cell therapy, GH3, and nutrition were included. It also described how to start your own life-extension program, and how to obtain hard-to-get nutrients and drugs.

Recently, the editors of Ronin Publishing obtained the rights to SOL with the intention of updating it. That update is still forthcoming, but in the meantime they have created this book entitled *Fountains of Youth,* an accessible introduction for the lay person to the field of life extension.

Chapter One defines aging, and describes the fundamental differences in approach to aging of traditional gerontology versus those who prefer a more activist life-extension approach, from both scientific and philosophical points of view.

A brief history of anti-aging legend and science is covered in the second chapter, which includes an introduction to the life-extending properties of caloric restriction. Chapters Three to Six selectively discuss various theories of aging, with emphasis on caloric restriction (Chapter Three), cellular aging (Chapter Four), and the free radical theory (Chapter Five). Chapter Six is an overview of a number of theories, without clearly delineating which theories have been largely discounted (error-catastrophe and somatic mutation), and which are still viable (neuroendocrine, and DNA-repair). Chapter Seven is a system-by-system overview of physiological changes that occur with age.

Chapter Eight describes the concept of biological aging measurement as a means to evaluate the success (or failure) of interventionist regimens. It includes three levels of testing: (1) a battery of simple tests which can be performed at home for relatively little output in time and money; (2) a routine battery of standard tests which can be conducted in a physicians office–most of which are part of a routine physical examination; and (3) a more complex, sophisticated battery of tests which are most likely to be available only in a research institution. Chapter Eight was adapted from my book *Biological Aging Measurement: Clinical Applications* which is available through the Center for Bio-Gerontology, P.O.Box 11097, Pensacola, FL 32524.

Chapters Nine and Ten–"How to Live Longer and Healthier" are broken down into two phases. Phase I is health advice–information one should get in a high school or junior college hygiene class ("Don't smoke, eat a healthy diet, get plenty of exercise, see your doctor regularly, and reduce your level of stress"). Phase II Life Extension consists of the recommendation to eat less, in order to gain the life-extending benefits of caloric restriction, and a discussion of the potential future benefits to be gained from research with growth factors and mitogens.

I am disappointed that there is little mention of the studies which have demonstrated life-extending effects of a number of substances. For example, the MAO-B inhibitor, selegeline, as well as melatonin, pineal polypeptide extract, and phenformin have all demonstrated increased maximum life span in animal experiments. Furthermore, while dehydroepiandrosterone (DHEA) supplementation has not thus far resulted in life span extension of experimental animals, its administration in both animals and humans appears to normalize (restore to more youthful levels) a wide array of metabolic parameters. This will often improve the quality of life, if not its length. Other hormones were likewise not mentioned (with the exception of growth hormone, which was not favorably reviewed). I believe that virtually all aging males and females can benefit from an individually-prescribed "hormone cocktail" of essential *natural* hormones, in psychological doses, resulting in a normalized hormonal profile with little or no adverse effects. While life-extending effects of such individual hormonal replacement regimens have not been demonstrated, there is certainly enough strong data regarding enhancement of the quality of life to justify such a program.

A unique aspect of the book is Chapter Eleven, the "Life-Expectancy Calculation". This is an instrument which is used by Dr. Chad Everone, one of the book's major contributors, at his *Center for Infinite Survival* in Berkeley, California. The Life Expectancy Calculation uses actuarial and lifestyle data to determine potential remaining years of life, and focuses on various techniques that can be employed to increase the life expectancy.

Fountains of Youth is a good introduction to biomedical geron-tology and the life extension movement for the beginning life extensionist. The advanced life extensionist, however, will probably already know much of the information in this book.

Ward Dean, MD.
The Center for Bio-Gerontology
P.O. Box 11097
Pensacola, Florida 32524

FOREWORD

by Chadd A. Everone, Ph.D.

Consider the fact that we exist in a monumental surge of historical events. We are not today where people were only some 50 years ago - 1) factors influencing how long we live are more complex; 2) the problems of longevity are different and more difficult; 3) while our potentials for living longer are much greater. Of all the forces of change which will be impacting upon us as we proceed into the beginning of the 21st Century, a big paradigm shift will be represented by the life extension sciences, because that is where human nature will be improved at its most fundamental level.

Some years ago, around 1973, Dr. Timothy Leary made the following, extemporaneous remark in a brief but intense conversation. He said:

> "If you want to change the human condition,
> then you must first change human nature."

By human nature, he did not mean psychology, morality, governmental systems or any of the "software" applications. Rather, he meant the "hardware" - i.e., human biology in general and specifically the human nervous system, its histology and biochemistry. Timothy Leary's thesis was that our conditions are as much emanations of our morphology as our morphology is a fit to our conditions. In other words, if you improve the human physiology, the consequences would be to improve the human condition in all of its aspects - psychological, political, economic, inter-relational, ecological, etc. This idea has stayed with me over the years; and it helped direct the course of my own profession into the life extension sciences. I believe that major human progress can be made only after we overcome the main barrier of human nature - - our relatively short genetically fixed life-span.

A practical life extension enterprise can use a fairly direct strategy that might be called intelligent but aggressive incrementalism. A variety of procedures are well established which anyone can readily implement. These practices prevent disease and improve biological vitality, resulting in a 10% to 30% increase in life span. That could mean a decade or more of additional, quality life. While integrating those applications into our personal life-style we can start positioning for long-range survival. Among a variety of things, this involves work, associations, geography and politics. It is important to stay in touch with the scientific developments in life-extension, and to contribute to and help promote basic research. Refinements and breakthroughs will occur, which will bolster biological vitality and additional increments on a healthy life-span will be gained. With some luck and a lot of well directed hard work, big breakthroughs in regeneration biology may be realized soon enough for us to take advantage of them. What would have been science fiction not long ago is now a realistic scenario.

In order to help you apply this scenario to your own situation, we have provided a Life-Expectancy Calculation in Chapter Eleven. This is a simplified version of the calculation I use in the Foundation for Infinite Survival Life-Extension Program. You might begin your reading of this book by first completing the calculation so that, as you proceed through the material, you can interpret and organize it around your own applications. This calculation is revised periodically to incorporate current developments. You can write to us for a revised form or download it from our Internet site (see information below).

The material in this book is about the science of life extension and its practical applications. However, life-extension, is also a philosophical and psychological matter. This is not to say that changing your philosophy or attitude will slow your aging or extend your maximum life-span. Practitioners of all the philosophies, both esoteric and exoteric, still age at the same rate, are afflicted by comparable diseases and have a similar maximum life-span. But to effectively engage in a life extension enterprise requires a desire to live longer. That desire comes from how much one values *life* and *self*, and one's vision of the future. These are core issues of psychology and philosophy. Once you start making changes in your life-style, even simple changes, your perceptions and attitudes change. You will start reevaluating your circumstances and your circumstances will start evaluating you. A change in you causes a readjustment in your circumstances. That readjustment causes a change in the *gestalt*, which feeds back to induce further change in you.

I have come to the opinion that when we get involved in life extension we should be prepared to work on our minds and our value systems. The psychological, social, and ecological implications of life extension are extremely important, but are beyond the scope of this book.

I would like to thank Beverly Potter and Sebastian Orfali for undertaking the publication of this work and the great amount of skill and effort which that entailed. Further, I would like to thank them for allowing me to say what I have to say, pretty much in the way I want to say it. We are still in the "wild-cat" phase of life extension science, and there are many different schools of opinion. They had the difficult task of blending a great deal of diversity. For my part, I am very definitive and tend to be rather positive in my rhetoric.

I have been engaged in life-extension science since 1972 and have worked directly in virtually all relevant aspects: clinical applications with all kinds of people in different situations, animal experiments on life-extension agents, library research, conferences, government agencies, bio-tech start-up companies, etc. Being positioned here in Berkeley, I am directly in touch with much of the fundamental science which pertains to life-extension technology. One prominent example is the Human Genome Project at Lawrence Berkeley Laboratory. This multi-billion dollar research project, when completed in about the year 2000, will provide the molecular "language" of the complete human genetic structure. This will provide for a new approach to medicine, including biological regeneration by the induction of cell division, which is my personal long range plan. The Genome Project is only one facility at the university that is relevant to this work. Further, the surrounding communities contain about 40% of all the bio-technology start-up companies in the world. We are uniquely positioned for rapid technology transfer, which is a big advantage.

Then there is the general environment and ambiance. Berkeley is a rag-tag, helter-skelter, free-enterprise zone. While on my way to a lecture by a high-level military planner who is giving an over-view of the future strategy of America's military, I can stop by the table of an activists group who wants me to sign a petition against Mitsubishi's lumbering operation in the rain forest. There is nothing like a *laissez faire* environment as an incubator for creative work.

I have explored the various options and I have come to the belief that for me the best approach to the control of aging is "caloric restriction." I believe this approach is dictated by the laws of human biology, and there is sufficient scientific knowledge of where we have to go for the final breakthroughs. We are beyond the descriptive phase of this science and into the phase of implementing the critical-path-strategy. I have a kind of "get out of my way; I know where I am going" attitude, which may be abrasive to many. I recall Sebastian Orfali protesting: "but you just can't say there is only one approach." My response was: "maybe *you* can't say that, but I sure can." Obviously, I will not know if I am right unless and until significant biological regeneration is demonstrated. That is still only a theoretical possibility, as of this date. So, even though the other editors justifiably toned me down my rhetoric I am grateful that they let me have my say much of the time.

Finally, I am confident that you will find this book both interesting and informative. I hope that you use the information and actively participate in future developments. I firmly believe that if you put into practice some of the basic procedures which are presented here, they will enhance both the quality and length of your life, which is, above all, the chief objective.

Best wishes for a longer and healthier life.

Chadd A. Everone, Ph.D., Governing Trustee
Foundation for Infinite Survival, Inc.
P.O. Box 5875
Berkeley, California 94705
http://www.fis.org

PREFACE

The search for longer life and extended youth is ageless. Recent and forthcoming discoveries may bring dramatic increases in longevity. Thousands of scientists are devoting their efforts to understanding, slowing, and reversing the aging process. Millions of people are taking steps to live longer and better. Many of them will live beyond the age of one hundred and twenty years, traditionally regarded as the maximum limit of human life.

"Who wants to be that old?" you might ask. Not many would care to hang around if it means being "old" in the sense that we have come to know the word. But what if the aging process could be slowed down and perhaps even reversed? What if you could look and feel like thirty when you are fifty or sixty; like forty when you are seventy or eighty; and better than most people at fifty when you are ninety or a hundred? What if you could avoid the aches, ailments, depression, anxiety, energy loss, and mental and physical deterioration that happen to many people during what are supposed to be the "golden years" of life? In short, what if you could remain throughout those one hundred and twenty years in a state almost as vibrant as when you were young? Would you turn down the chance?

This book explores what science is learning about the causes and control of aging. It examines therapies that many people are currently using to preserve youth and extend their life span.

A Guided Tour

To understand why aging occurs and how it can be controlled, we will take a guided tour through parts of the body where aging is initiated. We will journey into the various levels of biological organization from the genes to the cytoplasm to different cell types, organ systems, and the homeostatic, cybernetic integrated systems that comprise the body as a whole. We will travel through the bloodstream to the immune system, the "Jekyll and Hyde" of the body that can so easily switch from savior to saboteur. We will explore the brain and cognitive functions as they change with time. And we will descend even further, into the world of molecules, where we can gain a simplified understanding of some of life's complex chemistry.

In our "fantastic voyage" some unfamiliar biological and chemical terms may be introduced. It is important to understand scientific terms in order to understand precisely what happens during the process of aging. The information is presented in language that any reader should be able to understand.

Search for the Fountains of Youth

Control over the process of aging may be possible. The first chapter, "What Is Aging?" defines and presents a biological background to understand aging. To clarify our subject even more, Chapter Two, "The History of Life Extension," provides a summary of the history of life-extension efforts. It is a fascinating story, involving a full range of types of people: wild mystics, obscure mathematicians, hustlers and shysters, high-level movers of civilization, and a host of quiet "bench" scientists who do the day-in and day-out "donkey" work of empirical data collection. There are so many people involved in life-extension research—in *Longevity, Senescence, and the Genome*, a recent book that reviewed one aspect of aging, the author Caleb Finch made reference to the work of almost *six thousand* other investigators whose research went back over the last century. This history will enable you to view the progression of thought, to give a basis for understanding current directions in life-extension science. Scientific means to ameliorate the causes and effects of aging is the ultimate goal.

The next two chapters look at two different viewpoints currently used toward triumph in the war against aging: gerontological and life-extension approaches. Gerontology is the scientific study of the causes and effects of aging and of means for controlling or ameliorating these causes and effects. Gerontologists are the scientists who pursue this study. Longevists are not necessarily gerontologists, but are individuals who attempt to apply to themselves current knowledge about the control of aging. It is primarily the longevist to whom this book is directed, but anyone with an interest in health and preventive medicine should find this book useful. Life-extensionists view aging as the underlying cause of most chronic diseases–diseases that cannot be avoided or their onset delayed until the aging process is brought under control.

Following chapters present theories of aging, discuss diagnostic procedures for measuring biological aging and general health, and provide instructions for creating individualized life-extension programs for anyone interested in attempting to extend their life. This book does not attempt to make an argument for the "goodness" or the "shouldness" of life extension. Some life-extension authors spend a great deal of effort to make a convincing case for the practice of life extension. Most people in the field have moved beyond that issue. The focus now is on how to get to where we want to go as expeditiously as possible.

Anyone who has been following the recent progress of gerontology is aware that the human species is at a unique moment in its history and evolution. Human beings, the longest-living mammals on Earth, are on the verge of artificially extending natural life span by 50 percent, perhaps by more. Scientists have succeeded in extending the life spans of laboratory animals by means of caloric restriction and several drugs, indicating that there is more than one cause of aging.

Some of these anti-aging approaches are drastic, risky, or at least disadvantageous for human application. Others are essentially safe, and even generally beneficial because they promote life extension by enhancing health. "Even if they do not add years to one's life, they can add life to one's years."

The life-extension movement is expanding rapidly. Many people are not waiting for government sanction or good science to prevail, and are embarking on their own life-extension programs. Some are using drugs improperly, from which they are either deriving little good or are unwittingly causing themselves harm. Anything—even a vitamin—can be abused. Unfortunately, information is confusing. Much of the scientific and medical establishment continues in blind opposition to the entire life-extension movement.

By reading this book the reader should become grounded in essential scientific principles of life extension. By following the guidelines described herein, one may overcome rampant misinformation and disinformation, reduce the risks of drug misuse, and hopefully derive some benefits from a life-extension practice.

By offering this book, we are not urging the reader to use illegal or improperly validated therapies. Our goal is simply to try to supply as much information as possible, so that those who already intend to practice life extension may profit from valid scientific knowldege.

The information and ideas presented here are a result of a team effort by Ronin editors, with help from Chadd Everone, Ph.D., and Ward Dean, M.D., who created a draft manuscript inspired by John Mann's book *Secrets of Life Extension* . This manuscript has then been extensively edited by Mary Lou Sumberg, Beverly Potter, Ph.D., Sebastian Orfali, and Ginger Ashworth. These people are responsible for this incarnation of *Fountains of Youth.*

—Editors of Ronin Publishing

TABLE OF CONTENTS

5 THE FREE-RADICAL THEORY OF AGING　　　　　　75

6 OTHER THEORIES OF AGING　　　　　　　　　　　99

7 AGING AND THE BIOLOGICAL SYSTEMS 109

8 TOOLS TO MEASURE AGING AND GENERAL HEALTH 137

9 PHASE I LIFE EXTENSION: REDUCING DISEASE 159

10 PHASE II LIFE EXTENSION: EXTENDING LIFE SPAN 173

11 THE LIFE-EXPECTANCY CALCULATION 181

LIST OF ILLUSTRATIONS & TABLES

LIST OF ILLUSTRATIONS & TABLES

LIST OF ILLUSTRATIONS & TABLES

WHAT IS AGING?

Aging is more complex than the date on a birth certificate reveals. A 50-year-old person could have the body of an 80-year-old, or the body of a 30- year-old, depending upon many variables. If aging is indeed a disease, then a cure could be found. When or if this cure is discovered depends upon much scientific research yet to be accomplished.

AGING: A TREATABLE DISEASE?

Is aging a disease, the disease of modern times? If so, aging may be treatable, like any disease. The idea of aging as a disease, however, is incomprehensible to many people. Unfortunately, this includes people for whom this idea might have particular importance–the medical profession, government leaders, and scientists.

A personal anecdote illustrates the argument that aging may be a disease. Robert, a corporate lawyer in a successful practice, led the life of a *bon vivant* in San Francisco in the 1980s. Until his 50th birthday he never thought much about aging. On the morning of that day he looked into the mirror, as usual, but this time his internal self-image suddenly caught up with his physical reality. In horror, he uttered out loud: "My god, I'm dying!" In fact, that is what aging is–dying–slowly, incrementally, but nonetheless dying. The probable physical attributes of aging, including muscle atrophy, osteoporosis, memory and hair loss, wrinkles and spotted skin, are just reminders that death is becoming closer.

Every person makes unique adjustments to the realization of the process of aging. My friend did not take it well. He vacillated between depression and overcompensation. Tragically and pathetically he burned out much faster than was necessary. This book will show you how to avoid this type of negative reaction to aging.

QUALITY OF LIFE

Life span is not the preferred unit of measure. . . . The number of years we live is not too important if they are miserable years; our goal is to live better longer.

—Richard A. Passwater
Supernutrition

DENIAL DOESN'T STOP AGING

Denial is a powerful coping device of the mind. If a situation is unpleasant or painful and there seems to be nothing we can do about it, we tend to deny its existence. Or we may speak of it in euphemisms, or pretend we do not care, or disassociate from it. But if we really want to solve a problem it must be dealt with head-on and pragmatically Denying the existence of senescence (the aging process) won't make it stop, or make death go away. Only when we understand what is actually going on can we devise a strategy, based on empirical evidence, to retard aging and prolong life.

HUMAN LIFE SPAN

The following chart demonstrates what gerontologists have been dealing with for a long time. It follows the life span of people born in the same year. Variations related to sex and race are relatively minor. The general phenomenon of death applies to everyone.

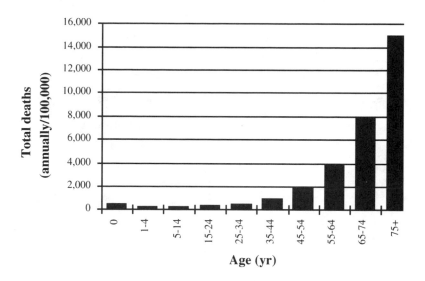

Figure 1.1 Aging Increases the Likelihood of Death
Data in this chart adapted by Chadd Everone from *Life-Extension Manual*.

This chart shows that when the incidences of death from all causes are graphed, there is an exponential increase in the death rate after about the age of 40. This acceleration of death is known as the "force of mortality." Gerontologists view this increase in the likelihood of death as being associated with or caused by aging or senescence. If the body had a constant structural integrity, and mortality were due only to the probability of accidents, infection, and other environmental factors, the chart would show a slow, linear increase in mortality over time even after age 40. Instead, it jumps exponentially. This means that the intrinsic structural integrity of the body is deteriorating as well as aggravating environmental injury. This same relationship to aging can be seen with the increase with age in the susceptibility to specific diseases.

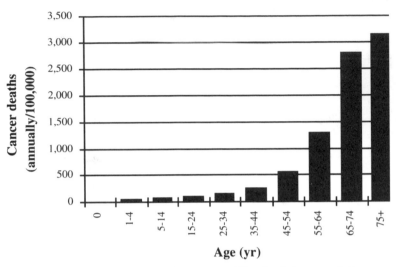

Figure 1.2 Aging Increases The Incidence of Cancer
Data in this chart adapted by Chadd Everone from *Life-Extension Manual.*

This chart shows that the incidence of cancer is also exponential with age and, therefore, is associated with or caused by aging. As some system or systems of the body break down intrinsically, cancers are more likely to occur. This is usually interpreted to be the aging of the immune system, and it could also be related to a decline in the accuracy of the repair, and replication of DNA, both of which are considered to be aging mechanisms. For example, the involution of the thymus gland, which happens at about age 20, dampens some aspects of the immune system. Concurrently, injurious chemical free-radical reactions from normal metabolism and from exposure to toxic substances cause damage to DNA, which causes cells to mutate. In an aging immune system, the probability of mutated cells veering off and spreading to other parts of the body as neoplasms or cancers becomes exponentially more likely. Thus, there is an increased risk of cancer with age.

This viewpoint, which serves as an introduction to the way geron- tologists think, highlights the fallacy of "conventional" medicine, which attempts to destroy cancer. Destroying cancer does nothing to restore the immune system, or buffer free-radical damage to DNA, or enhance the fidelity of DNA repair. In fact, two of the treatments for cancer–

chemotherapy and radiation–cause massive free-radical damage and hinder healthy DNA repair. It is possible that chemotherapy and radiation actually exacerbate the underlying conditions that caused the cancer in the first place. Perhaps that is why, even with the high-tech approach to cancer treatment, there has been little decrease in cancer mortality over the last sixty years.

HALFWAY THERE

Much of what is done in the treatment of cancer, by surgery, irradiation, and chemotherapy, represents halfway technology, in the sense that these measures are directed at the existence of already established cancer cells, but not at the mechanisms by which cells become neoplastic.

—Lewis Thomas
The Lives of a Cell

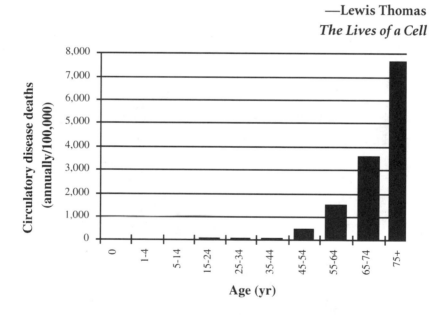

Figure 1.3 Diseases of the Circulatory System
Data in this chart adapted by Chadd Everone from *Life-Extension Manual*.

Heart attack, stroke, arteriosclerosis, and hypertension are associated with, and perhaps caused by, aging.

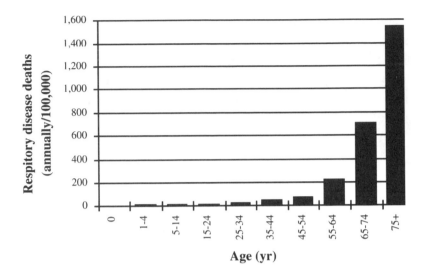

Figure 1.4 Diseases of the Respiratory System
Data in this chart adapted by Chadd Everone from *Life-Extension Manual*.

Diseases of the respiratory system are likewise associated with or possibly caused by aging.

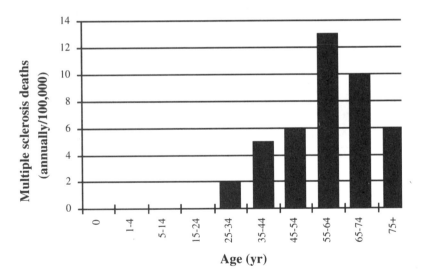

Figure 1.5 Multiple Sclerosis
Data in this chart adapted by Chadd Everone from *Life-Extension Manual*.

Not all diseases are related to the aging process. Multiple sclerosis, for example, is a disease to which only certain individuals are susceptible, either genetically or because of some accidental exposure to a pathogen. As the graph above shows, the incidence of multiple sclerosis does not increase exponentially with age; rather, it declines after age 64.

All of these data suggest the following: Biological aging could be viewed as a disease that operates beneath most of the recognized common diseases. If aging is cured, then other age-related diseases may also be cured. This perspective could dramatically alter the future of medicine and the human race.

ELIMINATE COMMON CAUSES OF DEATH

Let us explore some possible medical scenarios. Over one trillion dollars are spent annually in the USA on medical expenses. Let's assume that with this expenditure, medical technology could be taken to maximum efficiency. Now envision a situation in which instead of the 20 percent of the gross domestic product now devoted to medicine, medicine becomes to us what the pyramids were to the pharaohs, and 50 percent of our national income is devoted to this pursuit. Emergency crisis centers could be located in every neighborhood. Multiphasic checkups are regularly scheduled. At the slightest symptom, a diagnostic evaluation is performed. Everyone is instrumented with biological monitors with a telemetry system that feeds directly into the local crisis center. If a person feels faint or experiences any kind of pain, a medical team is immediately dispatched for emergency care. In this scenario, which is admittedly hyperbolic and facetious, there would be few deaths from cancer, heart disease, or the other common causes of death today. How much would you guess the average life span would be increased by such super-advanced technology? Look at the following table:

TABLE 1.6 THE ELIMINATION OF COMMON DEATH CAUSES RESULTS IN INCREASED LIFE EXPECTANCY

Cause of Death	Years Gained
Heart Disease	6.42
Cancer	2.23
Stroke	0.88
Respiratory Disease	0.69
Cirrhosis of Liver	0.28
Accidents Other Than Vehicular	0.28
Bronchitis, Emphysema, & Asthma	0.27
Influenza & Pneumonia	0.27
Vehicular Accidents	0.21
Diabetes	0.16
Atherosclerosis	0.10
Total Years Gained by Elimination of These Causes of Death	11.79

From *National Center for Health Statistics*

That's it! In a perfect medical world the average life span would be increased by only about twelve years, during which time everyone would progress into senescence and fade away in the convalescent home. This kind of medical world would be a complete personal, economic, and social catastrophe, unless aging were also controlled.

Aging also decreases adaptation to and recovery from stress. Millions of people over 65 currently require assistance with such routine acts of life as bathing and getting out of bed. Many millions more need aid with their finances, transportation, and meal preparation. Elderly people are increasingly less functional in social terms as well.

What therapies can be used to treat these consequences of aging? The problem of aging needs to be resolved. Let's look at current perspectives of aging from the gerontological as well as the life-extension viewpoints to see if a solution exists.

TREATING THE DISEASES OF AGING

There are two interrelated but different approaches to solving the problem of aging. One approach is to study the aging process; the other is to study life-extension models. Explaining the distinction between these two approaches can serve as an introduction to the basics of the science of longevity.

THE GERONTOLOGICAL APPROACH–AGING PROCESS

Gerontology is the study of senescence, the aging process. The goal of gerontological research is to discover which biological systems decline in vitality over time. The assumption is that once an accurate map is drawn of the systems that age, the underlying biochemical mechanisms–or primary aging mechanisms–can be identified. Corrective measures can then be invented to slow and/or reverse the degenerative process. Researchers seek to differentiate between a disease that afflicts only some individuals and the aging process that afflicts everyone.

Modern gerontological research began in the 1940s, which means more than fifty years of fairly concentrated investigation to study the primary aging mechanisms. Originally, researchers hoped to uncover one, or possibly a few, primary aging mechanisms. They postulated a "death hormone," or biological trigger, which causes the cascade of biological deterioration. This theory, however, has not been demonstrated. Within gerontology the death-hormone theory is now being replaced by a more complex model. The new theory holds that many or all biological systems age, in a process that differs somewhat in each individual.

The current status of gerontological research has been adequately summarized by some of the leading investigators from the College of Pennsylvania in Philadelphia.

STATUS OF GERONTOLOGICAL RESEARCH

Aging is an extremely complex biologic phenomenon of immense importance. Currently we have only a poor and incomplete understanding of the fundamental molecular mechanisms involved. Despite numerous observations and diverse theories, no unifying or proven hypotheses have emerged. It is reasonable to conclude, however, that aging is a multifactorial process composed of both genetic and environmental components. Each physiologic system within an organism, each tissue within a system, and each cell type within a tissue appears to have its own trajectory of aging. Thus, aging must be studied as parts of a whole and understood as the sum of its parts. Cellular "clocks" exist and operate in the absence of higher-order "clocks." However, higher-order clocks are certainly in place in vivo, but their relationship to cellular clocks is not well understood. All aging changes have a cellular basis, and aging is perhaps best studied, fundamentally, at the cellular level under defined and controlled environmental conditions. Aging changes at the cellular level must be viewed, however, as components of a hierarchical, dynamic, and interacting network whose functional integrity progressively deteriorates with time. The powerful tools of molecular biology are now being applied by scientists to evaluate the leading hypotheses. The results of these studies should serve to advance our understanding of aging and to focus future research efforts. This work should provide the scientific foundation to enhance the quality of life for people suffering the failings of age.

—V. J. Cristofalo; G. S. Gerhard; R. J. Pignolo

Molecular Biology of Aging
Surgical Clinics of North America

THE LIFE-EXTENSION APPROACH–WHAT SLOWS AGING

Research is also being done based on life-extension models. The goal of life-extension research is to study organisms in which the maximum genetic life span has been increased. Life-span extension is the criterion used to establish that biological aging has actually been slowed. In this situation, biological systems can be tested for aging, as in the gerontological model. Those systems which normally age, but in the life-extension model do not deteriorate, can then be judged as the primary mechanisms of aging. Those systems which decline, in the presence of increased life span, can be judged as secondary to the aging process. The use of life-extension models could resolve one of the central issues in gerontology: the issue of primary mechanisms. It could enable research to focus on the mechanisms of direct importance to the aging process.

THE DISTINCTION BETWEEN GERONTOLOGIC AND LIFE-EXTENSION APPROACHES

The distinction between the gerontologic approach and the life-extension approach may be difficult to grasp. However, it is a very powerful distinction.

Why is it important or useful to understand the technical aspects of life extension and the control of aging? What most people want to know is simply, "What should I do?" and "How much will it cost?" and "Is it certain to be effective?" In an established technology, that is the appropriate attitude. Life-extension technology, however, is still emerging. Because the experts disagree among themselves, it is necessary for the non-expert to understand the technical aspects. The rule of *caveat emptor*, or "Buyer beware" is the prevailing ethic in life-extension science at this time. The best consumer of products that enhance longevity is the one who is best informed.

SOME BASIC PRINCIPLES OF AGING

POLYMER CHEMISTRY & METABOLIC THEORIES OF AGING

The biochemistry of life is essentially the chemistry of polymers. The term "polymer" is a way of describing how a structural system is made. If something is a polymer, that means that it is a compound made from the linking of multiple, discreet units (Greek *poly*=many, *mer*=unit). A child's construction made from Lego® building blocks would be a kind of polymer–all the units are the same. But they can be put together in an infinite number of configurations to build almost anything conceivable. Genetic material is a polymer. The proteins that form your essential, structural material are polymers. Hormones and enzymes are polymers. Not all constituents of your body are polymers. Water, which constitutes most of the body weight, is not a polymer. Neither is fat nor glucose, the source of chemical energy.

Some standard tests used by many researchers, all the way from Nathan Shock, the grandfather of American gerontology, to award-winning scientist Roy Walford, will be presented in the next few pages in order to demonstrate some basic principles of aging.

This simple demonstration is a powerful experience. Do it mentally if it is inconvenient to do right at this moment–you will get the point. Obtain a photograph of yourself that was taken between the ages of 15 and 25, the chronological zone in which a human is developmentally optimal. During this segment of life, risk of debilitating disease or death is low; physical performance is at its peak. Ability to deal with stress is highest, and ability to recover from that stress is fastest. Your photograph reflects the ultimate expression of your specific, individual genetic composition. To recover and maintain the biological condition reflected in that image is the ultimate objective of life-extension and control-of-aging technology.

Take that photograph and paste it on a mirror. Juxtapose this youthful photograph with your present image. If you currently are 25 or 30 years old, you will probably not see much difference. If you are over 40, the difference in appearance will be distinct. As you grow older, it continues to become even more noticeable.

THE BIOLOGICAL STRUCTURE

What is happening to the underlying biological structure to cause these changes? Answering this question is the essential challenge of gerontology. If these changes can be described biologically in qualitative and quantitative terms, then it may be possible to elucidate the causes. If the causes of aging can be understood, then it may be possible to devise methods to slow the deterioration or restore youth.

With the mirror experiment, aging is seen at the level of surface appearance. To get an idea of aging at a deeper level, perform another experiment–the skin-elasticity test. Find a young person–under age 20. Each of you place one of your hands, palm down, on top of a table next to the other person's. Observe the differences in appearance. Next, gently pinch the skin on the back of your hand and pull the skin up, holding it for a brief moment. Then let it go. Notice the rate at which your skin returns to normal. Count the number of seconds to quantify this. Then do the same to the hand of the younger person. If you are 40 or older, you will observe that it takes your skin longer to return to normal than it takes for the younger person. The difference is caused by the dissimilarity in structural qualities of the skin at varying ages. What you saw was the result of deterioration in the matrix of the connective tissue. This is probably due to free-radical chemical reactions or limited cell-replication potential.

Deoxyribonucleic Acid (DNA)

When you look at your body, pull your skin, observe your breathing when exercising, feel your movement as you walk–even when you are reading this book and thinking–you are observing the reflection of a biological substrate and biochemical activity. You are a very ancient biological machine. You have ascended to this point in time from an unbroken chain of life forms that date back to simple origins on this planet some four billion years ago. The complexity of your body and the evolutionary process appear to be unfathomable. But now we know that this complexity is a reiteration of and variation on a genetic template called deoxyribonucleic acid (DNA).

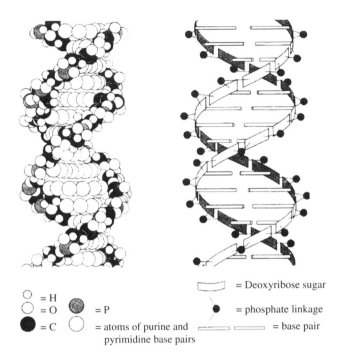

○ = H
○ = O   ◉ = P
● = C   ○ = atoms of purine and
              pyrimidine base pairs

▭ = Deoxyribose sugar
● = phosphate linkage
▭▭ ▭▭ = base pair

Figure 1.7 Deoxyribonucleic Acid
Graphic representation of DNA.
From *Introduction to Cell Biology* by Stephen Wolfe. Used by Permission.

DNA is a polymer of four simple base molecules. A polymer is a chemical compound formed by a chemical reaction in which two or more molecules combine to form larger molecules that contain repeating structural units. Originally, some four billion years ago, these molecules configured themselves into a master molecule that had the capacity to duplicate itself and to assemble other, supporting molecular structures. Of all mysteries, the origin of DNA is one of the most profound. We know that all life forms on the planet are made from this same molecule. DNA is the essence of you, the elephant, the plants in your yard, the mosquito that feeds on you at night, the virus that gives you the flu. You were made by your parents, who, in turn, were made by their parents, and on and on. All life forms come from prior life forms, which is to say from the old, original DNA. It is possible that, in the very beginning, there was only one DNA molecule that was made by accident. Thereafter it started "feeding" off of environmental materials, generating copies of itself, and making its constituent parts.

The propensity of DNA is to make exact copies of itself. In the process of replication, however, sometimes mistakes are made–mutations occur. Almost all mutations are maladaptive and die. A very few "fit" the environment. A mutation that adapts survives, reproduces, and proceeds on its own separate evolutionary path. Over the course of time, it is astounding how many variations DNA has made. A plethora of different life forms has been created. All of these life forms except the ones that exist today have become extinct.

The Cell

In the course of the history of DNA, one of the big evolutionary leaps was the invention of the cell.

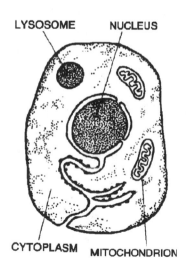

Figure 1.8 Simplified Animal Cell
From *Secrets of Life Extension* by John Mann. Used by permission.

The cell is a living unit, a small factory of many components. When you look at your body or stretch your skin, you are observing a hierarchy of biological systems, all of which are based on the cell as the main functional unit. Aging also occurs in the cells.

The cell is a composite of life forms. In the above graphic there are a number of small, cellular organs called organelles, located outside the nucleus of the cell. One of the organelles is called the mitochondrion. The mitochondrion has its own separate set of DNA, independent of the main, genetic DNA in the nucleus of the cell.

It is possible that in our ancient evolutionary past an organism that used oxygen for energy "infected" our cell line. It has lived symbiotically with us ever since, making us aerobic, or "oxygen-using," creatures. Human sperm, for example, has no mitochondria and uses a different, more primitive, anaerobic form of metabolism. Mitochondria are inherited from the ovum. Currently, certain aspects of oxygen metabolism are one of the main focuses of aging research. Oxygen metabolism is the central issue in the free-radical theory of aging, and the mitochondrion is a principal element in that discussion.

Anabolism and Catabolism

The cell is never static. Like an engine that cannot be turned off, the cell at least idles constantly. When subjected to increased stress, the cell automatically increases its metabolism. The essential metabolism of the cell involves active methods for constructing its elements (anabolism) and active methods for destroying its elements (catabolism). The cell is not like an ordinary manufacturing unit that makes its products only on demand. Since the cell does not know when there will be an increased demand, it must continuously manufacture its products in anticipation of a demand. If the cell's products are not needed it breaks the surplus units back down into basic components and proceeds to remake them. Like a gyroscope, the cell must always keep itself revving at a fairly high rate. This constant level of activity allows the cell to accommodate abrupt changes as well as ordinary demands without destabilizing its balance.

It is in this constant metabolic cycle of anabolism and catabolism that much of aging occurs.

Energy

Most of what a cell does is to make or remake its proteins. To do that requires the transformation of energy from sugar. At the most fundamental level, all living organisms derive their energy from sunlight. The sun bombards the planet with high-energy photons. Photosynthesizing algae and plants use the energy photons from the sun to combine carbon dioxide (CO_2) and ammonia (NH_3) from the atmosphere, water (H_2O) from the hydrosphere, and various minerals from the lithosphere. From those constituents, plants form proteins, fats, and sugars, and they release oxygen. Animals, such as ourselves, cannot convert the energy directly from the sun into usable energy like proteins, fats, and sugars. Animals consume plants or other animals that feed on plants in order to make use of the sun's energy. This is a complex and well-understood process.

The aspect of metabolism relevant to life extension involves the mitochondrion, which utilizes oxygen and water and a simplified sugar called pyruvate to synthesize adenosine triphosphate (ATP). ATP is the main energy molecule that enables the body to produce its polymers—vitamins, proteins, hormones, and enzymes. In the process of this energy conversion and synthesis of polymers, chemical by-products called "free radicals" are generated. Free radicals are the basis for one of the main theories of aging. (See Chapters Five and Six, which discuss the free-radical theory of aging as well as other contemporary theories.)

The next chapter, "History of Life Extension," discusses research already done from ancient times to modern times, which demonstrates how the past is a vital link to the present.

CHAPTER TWO

THE HISTORY OF LIFE EXTENSION

*T*he history of human endeavors to extend life and to control aging
is long, convoluted, and fascinating. The story includes a full range of
characters, from scoundrels to saints, and it depicts the evolution of human
consciousness from its earliest beginnings.

This chapter provides a condensed history of life extension, from myth
to folk medicine to the modern science of gerontology, the study of the aging
process. This background will place in perspective present theories of aging
and the scientific discoveries that have brought the science of life extension
to its present stage.

THE HISTORY OF LIFE EXTENSION
PARALLELS WITH THE HISTORY OF FLIGHT

A good analogy exists between the history of life extension and the
history of aviation. Since the earliest formation of consciousness, humans
have desired to fly. Over time, this desire gradually moved out of the realms
of myth and superstition into full realization. For both primitive and
modern humans, flying has symbolized power, freedom, the chance to see far
and wide, and the means to get to places fast. In order to capture that feeling
of power our primitive ancestors used what was available to them–their
imaginations and sympathetic magic. They wore eagle feathers, and they

carved images of the raven into tribal totem poles. They created mythic stories such as the Greek tale of Icarus, who donned wings made by his father and flew off into the sun. Archetypes of angels and cherubim have been depicted as winged beings throughout human mythology.

Modern humans have used science to capture that feeling of power. They learned some of the laws of physics and invented contraptions to capture the forces of lift and propulsion. Leonardo da Vinci designed mechanical wings similar to those of a kite or a bird. The internal combustion engine was linked to a winged vehicle and, with the Wright brothers, rudimentary flight actually began. Now hundreds of millions of people routinely fly through the air, faster and higher than anyone could ever have imagined. Beyond the airplane, Robert Goddard invented the liquid-fuel rocket. A generation later, a few of us have even jogged, ridden dune buggies, and played golf on the Moon.

The natural tendency of human hope, imagination, and aspiration is to find realization. In the words of Paracelsus, a 16th-century German physician who was a key figure in the history of science and a player in the theory of life extension, "Resolute imagination can accomplish all things."

As in the history of flight, the history of life extension can be divided roughly into three categories: myth, folk medicine, and science. Using the previous analogy, we currently are beyond the earliest scientific discoveries of the Wright brothers and Goddard stages; "lift-off" has been achieved, and we are poised for an onrush of breakthroughs.

The categories of myth, folk medicine, and science frequently overlap. Some observations made centuries ago are direct precursors of work being done today. For example, Hippocrates, a Greek physician who lived circa 460–370 B.C., associated aging with the loss of heat. Currently scientists are studying the decline in metabolic rate as we age, which is evidenced by a decrease in the body's heat production. This probably reflects a decline in protein synthesis within the cells of the body, and most probably is one of the basic causes of aging. Hippocrates also recommended the practice of moderation in eating and drinking, and caloric restriction is another area of modern-day research which shows incredible promise in studies on health and longevity.

MYTH, RELIGION AND LEGEND

A basic human desire is to live a long life on this planet, not in some imaginary realm. Throughout history, humans have attempted to understand *why* death is inevitable. Many people have sought refuge in religion, while some have searched for ways to stave off aging and prolong physical life. Legend and history are filled with tales of this search. According to historian Gerald Gruman from the University of Massachusetts, these legends commonly follow one of three basic themes: antediluvian, hyperborean, and fountain themes.

The antediluvian theme is founded on the supposition that humans once had very long lives, which somehow have shortened because of reasons such as human decadence or the will of the gods. The hyperborean theme is the idea that somewhere on this planet are people who already practice secrets of life extension and live very long lives. The fountain theme is another favorite type of longevity legend, based on the premise that a special substance exists which causes rejuvenation or extension of life.

THE HUBRIS SYNDROME

A 5,000-year-old Mesopotamian legend, the epic of Gilgamesh, is an ancient life-extension story that has survived to this day.

QUEST FOR IMMORTALITY

Gilgamesh is a vigorous young king who treats his people tyrannically. To oppose him, the gods create a wild man of great strength named Enkidu. At first the two combat each other. Out of that struggle they become close friends. Together, they go crusading throughout the world. After many exciting adventures, one day the heroes go too far and violate divine law, killing a sacred animal and insulting a Goddess. As punishment, the gods cause Enkidu to become sick and die, which brings the despondent Gilgamesh to a profound realization of his own mortality.

Gilgamesh for Enkidu, his friend,
Weeps bitterly and roams over the desert.
When I die, shall I not be like unto Enkidu?
Sorrow has entered my heart.
I am afraid of death and roam over the desert . . .

Gilgamesh becomes obsessed with the desire to find the secret of immortal life. He finally succeeds by obtaining a plant that has the power to rejuvenate. Due to negligence, he loses the plant, (the serpent steals it while he sleeps) so he must become resigned to the fate of death.

Gilgamesh, whither runnest thou?
The life which thou seekest thou wilt not find;
(For) when the Gods created mankind,
They allotted death to mankind,
(But) life they retained in their keeping . . .

—Gilgamesh translation from Gerald J. Gruman
"A History of Ideas about Prolongation of Life"
Transactions of the American Philosophical Society

Notice a message of futility in the Gilgamesh story, that any transcendental pursuit (i.e., a pursuit of life extension that transcends natural life-span constraints) often seems to be attached to a strong phobia that resides deep in the subconscious of the human mind. For example, in the mythology of flight and the story of Icarus, against his father's warning Icarus took the wings made by his father and flew as high as he could. The wings melted from the heat of the sun, and Icarus fell to his death in the ocean. The message, obviously a metaphor about transcending limitations, is clearly that it is precarious to do so.

It seems that we are held in check by an internal sense of *hubris* (the Greek concept that over-reaching pride brings punishment from the gods) about trying to become something which we are not. There is a little voice inside that seems to say: "You are what you are because that is the way you were intended to be; otherwise, you would be different from what you are. If you try to be more than allowed, then you may insult and offend Makers and evoke their wrath."

ONLY THE GODS ARE IMMORTAL

But, as it is, harsh old age will soon enshroud you–ruthless old age which stands someday at the side of every man, deadly, wearying, dreaded even by the Gods.

—Hugh G. Evelyn-White
The Goddess Aphrodite denying her
lover Anchises's request for immortality
Hesiod, the Homeric Hymns and Homerica

Another example of the hubris syndrome is the biblical story of the fall of man, from the book of *Genesis.* It is still a governing metaphor in attitudes toward life extension as well as in western civilization. Many people know the part of the story that depicts God's wrath because Eve violated the injunction not to eat fruit from the tree of knowledge; but few remember the full story in which there was a second tree–the tree of life.

ETERNAL LIFE

Then the Lord God said: "Behold! The man has become like one of us, knowing good and evil; and now, lest he put forth his hand and take fruit from the tree of life also, and thus eat of it and live forever." The Lord God therefore banished him from the garden of Eden, to till the ground from which he was taken. When he expelled the man . . . he stationed the cherubim and the fiery revolving sword, to guard the way to the tree of life.

—*Genesis 3:22–24*

THE INEVITABILITY OF DEATH IS THE
FOUNDATION OF MANY RELIGIONS

Aging and the inevitability of death are central elements in the metaphors that guide human civilization, particularly the religions. The Hindu prince Siddhartha Gautama ventured out of his protected life in the palace and proceeded to have four experiences that shaped his destiny. The first was the sight of an old, bent, decrepit man leaning on a staff. Siddhartha asked his charioteer what had happened to the old man. The charioteer explained that the man was old and that all men are subject to old age if they lived long enough. Next Siddhartha saw a sick man who was suffering from disease. Then he saw a dead man. The final experience was seeing a man who wore the yellow robe of a seeker and possessed serenity amid the dead, the diseased, and the aged. As a result, Siddhartha left his sheltered life and went out to live in the world. Eventually he became enlightened and founded the practice of Buddhism by which one can move through the travails of existence and still experience bliss.

Religions can be seen as doctrines of salvation constructed within an existential situation of inevitable suffering and death. The reasoning is simple: If earthly existence is futile, then beyond earthly existence there might be a realm of permanent beauty, happiness, pleasure, and eternal life. The challenge is to live this life in such a way that one gains access to the blissful life after death. The pursuit of a long life in the physical world has been associated with approximating spiritual perfection in the next world. Haunted by the brevity of earthly existence, humans have fabricated elaborate institutions to convince themselves that some sort of life continues after this one. As John Mann says in *Secrets of Life Extension* "Mesopotamians constructed ziggurats, pharaohs fashioned pyramids, and Christians built cathedrals reaching to the heavens, and all were aiming for the same thing. If eternal life could not be had on Earth, a compromise might be made for immortality beyond the grave." The idea of an afterlife, however, has not always been held with absolute confidence, and it cannot be proven.

THE ANTEDILUVIAN THEME

The antediluvian theme is based on the premise that in the ancient past humans lived very long lives. In western civilization, the Jewish, Christian, and Islamic patriarchs are depicted as having exceptionally long life spans.

TABLE 2.1 LIFE SPANS OF RELIGIOUS PATRIARCHS

Patriarch	Age at Death
Adam	930
Seth	912
Enosh	905
Kenan	910
Mahalalel	895
Jared	962
Enoch	365
Methusaleh	969
Lamech	777
Noah	950

From *Genesis 5:5–28, 9:28.*

These reputed life spans of the patriarchs have often been used to validate the pursuit of longevity. In 1267 Roger Bacon, one of the founders of the experimental approach to understanding nature, and a life-extensionist himself, believed that the average life span had been accidentally shortened and could be extended.

Why was I born if it wasn't forever?

—George Ionesco

PROLONGATION OF LIFE

The possibility of the prolongation of life is confirmed by the consideration that the soul naturally is immortal and capable of not dying. So, after the fall, a man might live for a thousand years [i.e., Methuselah]; and since that time the length of life has been gradually shortened. Therefore it follows that this shortening is accidental and may be remedied wholly or in part.

—Roger Bacon
Opus majus

Five centuries later, Benjamin Franklin wrote a letter to Joseph Priestley, the discoverer of oxygen, describing his vision of a future in which science had cured disease and extended the normal life span beyond that of the ancient patriarchs (the antediluvian standard).

BEYOND THE ANTEDILUVIAN STANDARD

The rapid progress true science now makes, occasions my regretting sometimes that I was born so soon. It is impossible to imagine the height to which may be carried, in a thousand years, the power of man over nature. We may perhaps learn to deprive large masses of their gravity, and give them absolute levity, for the sake of easy transport. Agriculture may diminish its labor and double its produce; all disease may by sure means be prevented or cured, not excepting even that of old age, and our lives lengthened at pleasure even beyond the antediluvian standard.

—Benjamin Franklin
Personal correspondence to Joseph Priestley

Ascending from Our Ancestors

The notion of our ancient ancestors living to such great lengths is considered a mythic construction. As far back as it goes, archæological evidence of the skeletal remains from our ancestors, shows that most of the earliest humans did not live much beyond the age of 40; the great majority died before 20. Consider that Stonehenge and the Great Pyramids were constructed mostly by teenagers. In the civilizations of ancient Greece and Rome, the average life expectancy was only 20 years. Since then, human life expectancy has remained about the same length, slightly improving over the years, until New England of 1750, when life expectancy was about 34. By 1900 life expectancy had reached about 47, and today about 70. In this regard we are not "descending" from our ancestors but rather "ascending" from them.

"Average Life Expectancy" vs. "Maximum Life Span"

Note that the term "average life expectancy" has been used, which is not the same as the "maximum life span."

Life Expectancy: the number of years a person *will probably* live

Life span: the maximum number of years a person *can* live

Over the millennia the *maximum life span* has remained fairly constant at about 100 years, but until recently few have reached that potential. Now, however, the *average life expectancy* has been extended to the point where most of us are approximating that potential. The distinction between average life expectancy and maximum life span is critical.

THE HYPERBOREAN THEME

The hyperborean theme consists of the idea that a human population already exists that knows the secrets of life extension and practices them, and thereby lives very long lives. This theme is based on the Greek legend of the Hyperborean tribe (*hyper*=beyond; *Boreas*=the north wind), a people who lived somewhere "beyond the north wind" whose life span averaged a thousand years.

HYPERBOREANS

...their hair crowned with golden bay-leaves they hold glad
revelry; and neither sickness nor baneful eld mingleth among that
chosen people; but, aloof from toil and conflict, they dwell afar...

—Pindar

Quests for Fountains of Youth

One famous life-extension quest was that of the aging, 16th-
century conquistador Juan Ponce de León. He began his career as an
explorer in 1493 as part of Christopher Columbus' second expedition to
the New World. One of his accomplishments was the founding of
Puerto Rico's oldest European settlement. Intrigued by a legend from
Bimini Island in the Bahamas about a "fountain of youth," and in pursuit
of new lands for the Spanish crown, he discovered Florida in 1513 As
John Mann quips in *Secrets of Life Extension,* "Instead of discovering
youth, Ponce De León discovered what is now the world's most extensive
old folks home!"

The quest for youthfulness continues today. Millions of people
make pilgrimage to Lourdes, in France, to experience the alleged mi-
raculous qualities of the water from an underground spring. And many
more people are searching for their own "fountain of youth" by ingesting
substances or applying therapies they hope will cause rejuvenation or
life extension.

MODERN MYTHS

Myth, or the psychological need for it, never dies. It just reconfigures
itself to fit a changed cultural environment. A current mythic genre is
science fiction, reuniting fantasy and science. Life extension is a
common and important theme in science fiction. Modern authors,
from Kurt Vonnegut to Anne Rice, have chronicled characters possessed
with immortality. A classic novel by Robert Heinlein, *Time Enough for
Love,* is a sweeping portrait of an individual who lives hundreds of years.

In this story, Heinlein explores important psychological, social, and environmental scenarios relevant to individual survival over an extended period of time.

The film *Blade Runner*, based on Phillip K. Dick's novel *Do Androids Dream of Electric Sheep?*, is a piece of sci-fi dealing with the quest for life extension. In this story, Dr. Elden Tyrell of the Tyrell Corporation designs and makes advanced "replicants" called Nexus 6. In every respect the replicants appear to be human. Dr. Tyrell has even implanted early childhood memories allowing the replicants themselves to think that they are human. The replicants are superior to humans in terms of intelligence and strength. Because of the concern that replicants might become a danger to society and the power structure, they are programmed for a short life span and banished to extraterrestrial worlds. A small group of replicants come to realize that they in fact are not human and that they have been programmed for an early demise. They go back to Earth looking for their maker to correct the defect. The epic scene is when Roy, the chief replicant, asks Tyrell if he can prevent them from dying at their predesignated time.

The dialogue that follows could have been constructed by some sophisticated scientific consultants in genetics, because the ideas are a plausible solution to aging. Tyrell proves to Roy that the termination sequence, once activated, cannot be reversed. He tries to console him by saying, "A light that burns twice as bright burns half as long." In grief and resignation, Roy gently embraces his maker, then viciously strangles him to death—a fitting revenge upon a creator who would deliberately cause to die that which he created! Unlike the myths of our ancestors, however, who seem to be more accepting of fate, the contemporary attitude is neither placid nor obeisant.

FOLK MEDICINE TRADITIONS

Since the beginning of recorded history, all kinds of herbs, waters, aromas, rituals, and practices have been used to cure disease and extend life—and the effectiveness of much of this folk medicine is supported by contemporary studies! For example, Hippocrates wrote in his medical aphorisms "in old persons the heat is feeble," an accurate description by modern standards of the decline in metabolic rate that characterizes aging. Aristotle, who lived circa 384–322 B.C.., expanded on this theme in his treatise *On Youth and Old Age, On Life and Death, On Breathing*, by linking respiration and dehydration to aging. Those two notions, expounded more than 2,000 years ago, are still a part of modern gerontological research. Third-century medical texts of the Sasanid Dynasty of Persia describe disease as originating from six basic causes: "Stench and dirt, heat and cold, hunger and thirst, anxiety and old age." Many people think that linking aging and disease is a new concept, when actually the link is ancient.

LONGEVITY TRADITIONS FROM THE ORIENT

The Chinese people have a long tradition of interest in longevity and the search for methods to gain it. Legends exist of the *hsien*, immortal people who live forever because of their mastery of longevity techniques. Taoism, the central religious philosophy of China since 200 B.C.., has among its goals life extension and physical immortality.

THE TAO OF LONGEVITY

Who eats the elixir of life and guards the One (Tao), lives as long as heaven exists, he revives the constituents of his nature, stores up his breath, and thus lengthens his life indefinitely.

—Ko Hung
Pao-p'u Tzu

Taoism is a complex philosophy that combines religion, magic, mystical notions, and proto-science. Life-extension practices have always been a prominent feature of the Taoist system. Four techniques have been used to increase longevity; upon perfection they bring physical immortality to the practitioner.

1. Breathing techniques, that link the body to the external divine spirit
2. Dietary techniques that limit food intake to a bare minimum (caloric restriction)
3. Exercise techniques called *kung fu* (a form of martial arts involving all the muscles of the body)
4. Sexual techniques involving *coitus reservatus* (avoidance of male orgasm)

To this day, these practices are used in various systems of health and esoteric psychology.

LIFE-EXTENSION FOLK PRACTICES

In Secrets of Life Extension, John Mann gives Thomas Parr as an example of the benefits of dietary restriction: "This English peasant is reputed to have lived for more than a century and a half, sustaining himself on a frugal diet of fruit, cheese, and black bread. In 1635 he was brought before the court of King Charles, where he was lavishly wined and dined by those who hoped to learn his secret, and soon he died of overindulgence! An autopsy showed Parr's supposed 152-year-old brain and organs to be in a marvelous state of preservation."

Another life-extension practice was described by Cohausen in 1771 in his work *Hermippus redivivus: or the sage's triumph over old age and the grave. Wherein a method is laid down for prolonging the life and vigor of man. Including a commentary upon an ancient inscription, in which the great secret is revealed, supported by many authorities.* Cohausen, in his study of mediæval manuscripts, discovered the following arcane inscription:

> L. CLODIUS HERMIPPUS
>
> Lived one hundred and fifteen years and five days
>
> by breath of young women, which
>
> is worthy of the consideration
>
> of physicians and of posterity.

In pursuit of longevity, Cohausen spent a fair portion of his life compiling evidence from historical documents to support the case that there is some essential vapor in the respiration of young virgins that has rejuvenating power. Apparently this was a practice which, in Cohausen's words, was "a certain medicine concealed by wise men, least the incontinent should offend their Creator." Millennia earlier, physicians reputedly prescribed this same treatment to provide warmth and prolong life for the ailing King David, written about in the Old Testament (*I Kings* 1:1–4).

Recently scientists have discovered chemicals called "pheromones." These chemicals, apparently emitted by individuals, induce biological response in other individuals. This is not far removed in concept from the vapors of Cohausen. However, any ability of pheromones to rejuvenate the old is probably fanciful.

The pursuit of life extension did not stop at those relatively innocuous tinkerings, but became more aggressive with the approach of 20th-century medicine.

THE MODERN SCIENCE OF LIFE EXTENSION

It is not so much that science is separate from myth or folk medicine–rather, it is a refinement of those intuitive faculties. What characterizes modern science is two things: first, the careful gathering of relevant and accurate facts (reproducible data); and second, controlled experiments using models or integrated theories of reality as a basis for understanding the mechanisms of natural phenomena. Once such an understanding is gained, a scientist can accurately *describe* events and *predict* outcomes. Good science is painstaking intellectual and physical work, usually low on the scale of fame and fortune. It takes sustained effort over a long time.

THE EFFECT OF 19TH-CENTURY
RESEARCH ON MODERN GERONTOLOGY

Charles Edouard Brown-Sequard, born in 1817, was a precocious student. He graduated as a doctor in Paris at the age of 23 and then studied experimental medicine at Harvard. In 1859 he migrated to England and became physician to the National Hospital for the Paralyzed and the Epileptic. Five years later he was back at Harvard as Professor of Physiology and Nervous Diseases. He subsequently returned to Paris as a professor at the École de Medicine, next traveled to New York again, and then came back to Paris. In 1878 he succeeded the great physiologist, Claude Bernard, as Professor of Experimental Medicine in the College de France, a position he maintained until his death.

Brown-Sequard's medical research was fruitful. He confirmed Claude Bernard's work on the sympathetic nervous system, provided valuable knowledge of the effects of arrangement of the nerve fibers in the spinal cord, and conducted important experimental work on the subject of epilepsy, as well as studies on heat exhaustion and the nervous system. He also had the distinction of founding and editing two learned medical journals—the *Journal de la physiologie de l'homme et des animaux*, which was published from 1858 to 1863; and the *Archives de physiologie normale et pathologique*, which he founded in 1868 and produced until his death. He wrote nearly five hundred scientific papers during his lifetime.

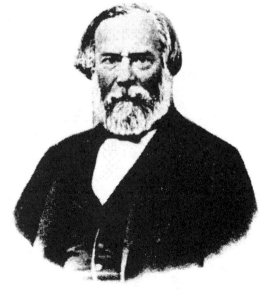

Figure 2.2 Charles Edouard Brown-Sequard
From *Secrets of Life Extension.* Used by Permission.

THE WORK OF BROWN-SEQUARD

For most of his life, Brown-Sequard was regarded as a distinguished scientist with an untarnished reputation. Toward the end of his life, however, an event occurred that was to lead to his professional downfall. Prior to his 70th birthday, Brown-Sequard began conducting dynamometer tests on himself to observe in experiments the effects of age on muscular strength. He had also begun to suffer from fibrositis, fatigue, and sleeplessness. He began by injecting himself with extracts made from the testes of small animals. The results were apparently startling. He found himself surprisingly rejuvenated, sexually, and with increased muscular strength as demonstrated with the dynamometer.

On June 1, 1889, Brown-Sequard made a presentation at a meeting of the Société de Biologie that was world-shattering in its conception. Holding a small vial of fluid in his hand for all to see, he disclosed that he had made an extract of animal sexual glands and that although he had had only three injections of it so far, he was tremendously rejuvenated. Brown-Sequard had married recently (for the third time), and was proud enough to boast to the assembled audience that he had been able to satisfy the young Madame Brown-Sequard after the injections. This added spice and sensationalism to a meeting that had gathered presumably to hear a cold and serious scientific paper.

Brown-Sequard must have looked as young as he alleged he felt (i.e., thirty years younger) because the popular French papers jumped on the news with alacrity. *Le Matin* immediately proposed to erect an Institute of Rejuvenation where the "Sequardian Method" was to be practiced for the benefit of aging Frenchmen. Brown-Sequard and his assistant, d'Arsonval, invented a fantastic "Rube Goldberg" type of machine with a belt, pulley, tubes, aeration bladders, and instruments. Into the machine they fed bull testes, pulped, filtered through sand, and ascepticized with boric acid. They drew off the resulting solution, and injected it into the buttocks of aging Frenchmen. Unfortunately, the commercial preparation from bull testes did not seem to have the positive effect on the general populace that the laboratory-produced version had on Brown-Sequard. It has been suggested that the method used for the mass extraction of testes was the reason for its inefficacy.

Popular support for the Sequardian Method collapsed. The medical profession was in vehement opposition. Apart from a paper he published in 1892, in which he argued that the kidney produced an internal secretion (later confirmed), he published no further work. His young wife deserted him, and he died on the Riviera of a stroke in 1894, at the unremarkable age of 77.

Not long after, a worse catastrophe occurred in the development of life-extension science. Dr. Serge Voronoff was a dapper, effervescent physician who was every inch a stereotype of a medical rejuvenationist. He believed that aging was associated with "testicular exhaustion or deficiency." His solution was to transplant ape testicles to men. He performed several hundred operations, actively seeking publicity in the newspapers to recruit new patients. Unintentionally, Voronoff infected many of his patients with syphilis from the monkeys. The infected patients died horrendous deaths.

Both Brown-Sequard and Voronoff were respectable medical researchers, but the allure of rejuvenation can have such a strong emotional appeal that good judgment and caution are sometimes abandoned. They represent good examples of "look before you leap." Although they suffered humiliating downfalls, all was not lost. Their work pointed in a valid direction, and their attempts stirred others into a more active search for a glandular key to rejuvenation. Life-extension science was, however, traumatized by these episodes. These catastrophes probably set back progress in the field for decades. Ever since, life extension has carried a connotation of quackery. Because of this, most professional gerontologists still distance themselves by insisting that their aim is not life extension but rather the *study* of aging.

THE FORCE OF MORTALITY

In a given population of humans, the likelihood of death
doubles about every eight years after age thirty, thus limiting the
maximum life span of humans to a defined number of years. This
is called the "force of mortality." The equation is $q_x = q_0 e^{alphax}$
(where $q_x = d_x/hL_x$ is the death rate at age x; d_x is the number of
deaths between age x and age x + h; L_x is the number alive at age x).

—Benjamin Gompertz

"On the Nature of the Function Expressive of the Law of Human
Mortality and on a New Mode of Determining Life Contingencies."
Philosophical Transactions of the Royal Society of London

THE FORCE OF MORTALITY

The clinical beginning of modern life-extension science and gerontology can be ascribed to an obscure English mathematician by the name
of Benjamin Gompertz. In the early 1800s, Gompertz traveled around
the countryside, recording birth dates and death dates from tombstones
and church records to see if he could derive a mathematical equation to
predict the probability of death. After years of meticulous data collection, he formulated a simple mathematical equation. This rule essentially states that after the age of 30 the risk of death increases exponentially with age.

One premise of gerontology is that aging is a disease, an inborn
genetic defect that has been inherited by all members of the species.
Gompertz's equation may support that premise. This phenomenon
applies to most vertebrates and to all mammals.

Later in the 1800s, with the advent of the germ theory of disease,
there was a brief period when it looked like all disease might be
attributed to specific germs and be curable by drugs or immunization.
Louis Pasteur, the originator of germ theory, eventually had to conclude,
however, that loss of host vitality (i.e., individual health) rather than
germs was the most fundamental factor leading to disease and death.

TWENTIETH-CENTURY EXPERIMENTATION

In the early 1900s experimenter J. Loeb raised animals in "perfect" environments, i.e., with ideal temperature and nutrition, and completely sterile from infectious organisms. It was found that animals in perfect environments still died at the same rate and time as predicted by the Gompertz equation. It is this law that establishes the "survivorship curve."

SURVIVORSHIP CURVE

A survivorship curve is graphic representation of the number of individuals in a population that can be expected to survive to any specific age. There are three general types of curves. The first, characteristic of small mammals, fishes, and invertebrates, has a high death rate (or low survivorship rate) immediately following birth. The second type, illustrated by the larger mammals, is the opposite. The organism tends to live a long life (low death rate and a high survivorship rate). Toward the end of its life expectancy, however, there is a dramatic increase in the death rate. In the third type, found in birds and mice, the mortality or survivorship rate is relatively constant during the organism's entire life.

—*The New Encyclopedia Britannica*

The survival curve is important because it is the heart of life-extension science and the framework for determining the validity of claims of life extension and control of aging.

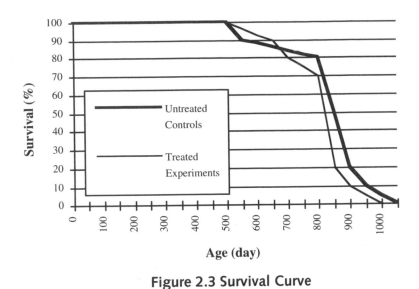

Figure 2.3 Survival Curve

Foundation for Infinite Survival, Inc., Life-Extension Program, Experimental Animal Colony

Above is a standard survival curve. On the vertical axis is the "percent surviving" and on the horizontal axis is the "span of time." A control group represents a group of subjects (usually animals, but it could be humans) that are maintained under normal living conditions. An experimental group is being given a therapeutic agent. The percent surviving is plotted over time.

If the therapeutic agent is effective in preventing disease there would be a slight shift to the right, in the survival of the experimental group. If the agent is effective in slowing or reversing aging, then a much more dramatic shift to the right will occur in the experimental group. As can be seen in the above experiment, which involved the administration of thyroid and an insulin-promoting factor, there was no life extension. The experimental agent was ineffective, both in preventing disease and in slowing aging.

THE AVERAGE AND MAXIMUM LIFE SPANS

A corollary to the survival curve is the fact that there is a fixed maximum life span that is characteristic of each species. To change that, one must alter the intrinsic aging of the system. See the table below for some examples of maximum life spans.

TABLE 2.4 EXAMPLES OF LIFE SPANS

SPECIES	AVERAGE LIFE SPAN IN MONTHS	MAXIMUM LIFE SPAN IN MONTHS
Human	849	1380
Chimpanzee	210	534
Domestic Cattle	276	360
Goat	108	216
Horse	300	744
Elephant	480	840
Cat	180	336
Dog	180	408
House rat	30	56
Mouse	18	42

Data adapted from Rockstein, Morris, et al., *Handbook of the Biology of Aging*, Caleb E. Finch & Leonard Hayflick

EXPERIMENTAL MODELS

The second building block of scientific gerontology has been the development of animal models for the purpose of controlled experiments. The essential idea is to work with an animal that has all the organs humans have, as well as a similar kind and distribution of diseases. A relatively short life span is desirable so that the experimental results can be obtained in a reasonable length of time.

Fruit flies are inexpensive to maintain and have a life span of only about seventy days. They would be great experimental subjects if they were closer to humans in terms of structure and disease patterns. Biologically, chimpanzees are almost identical to humans, but they live a long time and are expensive to maintain. Rats are close to humans and, except for the fact that they continue to develop throughout most of their life span, they would be appropriate under certain conditions.

A commonly used life-extension model is a mouse. Mice have a short life span (average 1.5 years); they are inexpensive and easy to maintain; and they have a developmental sequence similar to humans. There are different kinds of mice. The standard for life-extension studies is the C57BL/6J mouse.

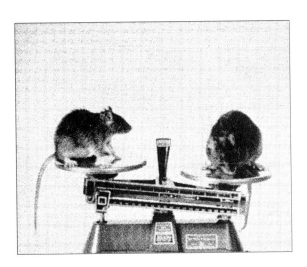

Figure 2.5 C57BL/6J Mice Used in Life-Extension Experiments
From *Secrets of Life Extension* by John Mann. Used by permission.

The ancestors of this mouse came from China hundreds of years ago, where the selective breeding of mice was an art form. The practice was picked up by the Japanese. When the British started trading with Japan in the late 1700s they too learned the Chinese technique for breeding mice. The ancestors of the C57BL/6J mouse came to the United States from Britain about 1920 for cancer research. This mouse strain was further developed by Jackson Laboratories in Bar Harbor, Maine. Since 1951 this strain has been maintained for aging research by the National Institutes of Health.

The "C57 blacks" are easy to obtain for scientists doing life-extension experiments. If a researcher gets a significant extension of maximum life span in the C57BL/6J mouse, then the scientific community will know what that means and whether the results are valid and relevant. There is a long history and large allocation of time and resources that support the development of proper animal models for experimental research.

Biological Parameters—"Biomarkers"

The third basis of modern scientific life extension is the development of "biomarkers," which are measurement parameters of aging.

The use of biomarkers in the measurement of human aging had an incongruous beginning. After the atomic bomb was dropped in World War II, individuals who had been subjected to large amounts of radiation appeared to be aging at an accelerated rate. In the late 1940s a team of scientists from Yale University was commissioned to study these people. The parameters originally tested were relatively simple and included such factors as cholesterol, blood pressure, exertion, hearing, and vision. This work was greatly expanded by Nathan Shock in the Baltimore Longitudinal Study, and it continues to this day. This is a complex field, and many issues remain to be resolved. It is currently the focus of many investigators throughout the world.

The essential idea behind biomarkers is the following: Life extension and control of aging matters to you only if *your* personal aging is being slowed and *your* life is being extended. In an experimental study on mice there was a correlation between the biomarker of serum glucose levels and longevity. Lower blood glucose than normal correlated with longer life span. However, although it is a good experimental model, the mouse is still remote from the human. Evidence from animals can be only inferentially applicable.

Clinical Studies

Next in the hierarchy of evidence is the clinical study. In a controlled clinical study on people a strong statistical correlation was found between lower glucose levels and length of life. However, a controlled study in a selected group of humans is not a controlled study in *you*. You need to know what your specific personal glucose level is and how to keep it in the low-normal range according to your biological individuality. Furthermore, you need to know if a low-glucose level is effectively slowing *your* aging, lowering *your* risk of disease, and increasing *your* life expectancy.

Over the past forty or so years, one of the central efforts of gerontology has been to find a battery of tests that measures aging in specific individuals within a fairly short period of time. Intervention techniques can then be tested on the individual person, where it is ultimately relevant. See Chapter Eight, "Diagnostic Procedures for Measuring Biological Aging and General Health," for some examples of available testing batteries to measure aging that have been designed by many research centers around the world.

BASIC RESEARCH ON AGING & LIFE EXTENSION

The final element in the scientific approach to life extension and control of aging is the experimental research that focuses on the basic biological aging mechanisms. There are two interrelated but different approaches. Theories of aging focus on the aging process. Theories of life extension focus on methods that slow aging and prolong life.

Most of the work has been done in the field of gerontology, which is the study of the aging process. The central belief of gerontology is that once it is understood which biological systems decline after the age of 30, then methods can be devised to slow or reverse that decline.

The problem has been that it is extremely difficult to discern which systems decline because of aging and which decline because of specific diseases. In the last stages of life, near the end of the maximum life span, virtually all systems have severely declined. However, it is not clear whether this is a cascade phenomenon in which the deterioration of a few primary systems causes the deterioration in general, or whether multiple systems decline simultaneously. The central dilemma with the gerontological approach is that there has yet to be one instance in which the backward correction of one system has significantly extended the maximum life span. The reason for focusing on maximum life span is that it cannot be changed unless the underlying aging has been affected.

CALORIC RESTRICTION

The other approach to the problem uses the life-extension model as its primary point of reference. Caloric restriction is a technique that has greatly extended the maximum life span in all species studied and will most likely do so in humans. Caloric restriction modifies biological aging and increases the maximum life span by 50 to 100 percent! When the biomarkers are studied in calorically restricted animals, one can see which systems continue to decline along the normal course and which systems are better maintained. Perhaps those systems that continue to decline are not the critical or primary ones; and those systems that are better maintained are the ones that are the leading mechanisms of aging.

AGING THEORIES

The people proposing aging theories remind me somewhat of the story of the seven blind men examining an elephant: to the one feeling a leg, an elephant is like a tree; the one feeling the trunk thought he was like a big snake, etc.; each being correct so far as he went. So with the aging theories, each is probably correct to a certain extent.

—Denham Harman
Robert Prehoda
Extended Youth

The leading theories of aging will be reviewed in upcoming chapters. Aging and its treatment should receive emphasis in medicine and health. This point of view is still not part of the standard medical philosophy nor the general conception of the public at large.

CHAPTER THREE

THEORIES OF AGING— THE LIFE-EXTENSION APPROACH

There are two interrelated but different approaches to solving the problem of aging. One approach is to study the aging process. The other is to study life-extension models. This chapter will focus on the life-extension model of aging as its primary point of reference. So far, there is definitely one technique that has greatly extended the maximum life span in all species studied (and will most likely do so in humans): caloric restriction. Caloric restriction modifies biological aging and can increase the maximum life span up to 100 percent!

The maximum life span of cold-blooded animals can be extended by slightly lowering their body temperature. Some types of trees live naturally for thousands of years. Single-cell organisms can live indefinitely, as long as the environment is hospitable. But those life forms are remote from mammals and not applicable to humans. Throughout the histories of medicine, hygiene, physical fitness, sanitation, and the study of biology and physiology in general, there has been only one method that has significantly extended the maximum genetic life span in experimental models relevant to humans.

ARE YOU INTERESTED IN
INCREASING YOUR LIFE SPAN?

Consider for a moment the following proposition. If you heard of a therapy that would improve your physical vitality by more than 20 percent and thereby increase your life expectancy by a good ten to thirty years, would you give it some serious attention? Suppose further that administering the therapy is completely within one's personal control, that it does not require any professional management or technology, and that it protects against cancer, heart attack, and a host of other chronic diseases, in the course of extending life span.

As a first step in incremental life extension, this therapy would be a very good start. Are you interested? There is yet another incentive: it costs you nothing. Indeed, you would save money and time. Remember the sayings "A penny saved is a penny earned" and "Time is money"? Taking into account the actual savings and, if you place a very modest monetary value on your time, your earnings could be twenty dollars per day.

Using some simple calculations, if you were to take that twenty dollars and invest it in a mutual fund and retain the earnings, over a period of ten years you will have earned about $55,000; in fifteen years, $170,000; in twenty years $500,000; and in twenty-five years over $1,000,000. This should be more than enough money to pay for complete genetic reengineering by the time that becomes an available technology, and then, have enough money left over to go out afterward and have some fun!

Increase in vitality, increase in life expectancy, decrease in risk to disease, able to implement on one's own, and earns money—does this sound too good to be true? Well, it is true! But chances are that your interest will rapidly evaporate when you find out that it involves eating about 40 percent less food than you normally do. Now, at this point, the sound of books slamming shut can be heard across the nation. But, before you abandon this subject altogether and toss the book in the recycling bin, read a little further—someday you may change your mind.

CALORIC RESTRICTION

This therapy is called variously "caloric restriction," "dietary restriction," or more currently, "energy restriction." Energy restriction is technically accurate because it is known that what is being restricted is the energy content of food and not specific nutrients. That term, however, connotes a lack of energy and a state of lethargy. These conditions do not occur, even though the amount of energy consumed in food is being restricted. In order to avoid that possible misinterpretation, the traditional term, caloric restriction, is used throughout this book.

Of the many attempts to increase longevity, caloric restriction is one that has increased the maximum genetic life span in mammals. It has done so dramatically—on some occasions, almost doubling it. No one in the scientific community would dispute this statement. Caloric restriction works in mice, rats, bats, hamsters, dogs, and cats. It works in insects, fish, and even microorganisms. After a century of research and several hundred controlled studies, caloric restriction has been shown to be effective in increasing maximum life span in virtually every case where it has been used.

INCREASED LIFE SPAN OF THE PEOPLE OF THE HUNZA

The people of the Hunza do not consciously follow any special diet...they eat two meals a day, drink glacier water, and mix work with exercise and pleasure. They do not contaminate their soil. Occasionally, they run out of food at the end of the winter season. Until the new crop is available they have practically nothing to eat, and water has to suffice. Apparently it nourishes them well and they easily survive the period of near starvation. We would call it fasting.

—Renée Taylor
The Hunza-Yoga Way to Health and Longer Life

Controlled studies using humans as subjects have yet to be accomplished. The people of the Hunza are an isolated group of people who practice caloric restriction by necessity and allegedly live remarkably long, healthy lives. Scientific verification is difficult to obtain, however, from societies that do not always use record-keeping practices such as birth certificates, but the average life span of these people is reputedly over a hundred years. By eating only two frugal meals a day and fasting for several weeks at the end of winter, these people are modern-day exemplars of caloric restriction.

CALORIC RESTRICTION ON PRIMATES

Caloric restriction is currently being tested in rhesus monkeys in order to evaluate its effect on primates. This study is being portrayed as the definitive study upon which caloric restriction can either be recommended for human use or disregarded as irrelevant to human aging.

It will be worthwhile to explore some of the particulars of this primate research to illustrate how some scientific projects come into being for reasons quite extraneous to the gathering of good and necessary information. There are some major problems with this study, and many scientists believe that a great deal of time, money, and expertise will be expended with nothing gained in terms of real knowledge.

First, primates live a long time. It will take more than twenty years to complete this research. If we wait for the final results before taking appropriate action, many of the scientists who are doing the study as well as the readers of this book will be either dead or in a convalescent hospital.

Second, caloric restriction works in all species tested thus far, including many different kinds of mammals. There is valid reason to assume that it will work in humans. If there were a valid rationale for suspecting the existing animal evidence on caloric restriction vis à vis humans, the same suspicion would hold true for other biomedical knowledge in which animal models have been used. This would cast doubt on almost all areas of medical research from toxicology to cancer, from infectious disease to surgical techniques. Caloric restriction probably will work in humans. Privately, most researchers know this. The primate study may be scientifically unnecessary, expensive, and take a long time. Why then is it being done? In great measure, in response to political pressure.

What happened was this. Edward Masoro, an important nutrition research scientist in the Department of Physiology at the University of Texas in San Antonio, has done a great deal of research on nutrition and life extension. He supports the idea that caloric restriction in other mammals is relevant to humans. In concert with Masoro, Roy Walford, a famous researcher at the University of California in Los Angeles, has advocated the same position and has taken caloric restriction in humans very seriously. Walford wrote a book in 1986 called *The 120-Year Diet*. More recently, he and his daughter have written another caloric-restriction book titled *The Anti-Aging Plan*.

Masoro and Walford have generated much publicity about and public interest in caloric restriction. As a result, the federal government's National Institute on Aging felt pressured into doing something. About the only thing left to do in the area of caloric restriction and life extension is a primate study.

D. K. Ingram proposed such a study. Some clues are given in the preliminary report on the proposed experiment, which has been funded by the National Institute on Aging.

TESTING CALORIC RESTRICTION IN ANIMALS

In light of the intense recent interest in the mechanisms, physiological validity, and possible applicability of dietary restriction to humans (Masoro, 1988; Walford, 1986), it has become essential that this phenomenon be tested in animal models more closely related to humans.

—D. K. Ingram
Proposal to National Institute on Aging

There is an important scientific criticism of the proposed Ingram study involving the experimental design, particularly the number and source of the animals. The following excerpt from the study methods depicts the problem:

NUMBER AND SOURCE OF EXPERIMENTAL ANIMALS

Male rhesus monkeys (Macaca mulatta) were acquired during December 1986–February 1987 and consisted of: 12 juveniles (0.6–1.0 yr. . .), 12 young adults (3–5 yr. . .), and 6 old (>18–25 yr. . .). Both juveniles and adults were born in captivity. . . . The juvenile monkeys. . .from the NIH facility in Perrine, Florida. . . . The adults. . .from the People's Republic of China. . . . The old group was captured in India. . . .

—D. K. Ingram
Caloric-restriction Study

One need not be a trained scientist to see problems with the number and source of experimental animals. There are only twelve juvenile animals, which means six controls and six experimentals; twelve adult animals, again six experimentals and six controls; and six older animals, which were captured in the wild to be used as "normals." How can any meaningful information come from such small numbers of environmentally diverse animals? Scientifically, there is nothing here to either refute or confirm Walford's and Masoro's claims. It would be better to use a group of humans as in the Framingham Study for heart disease, or the Baltimore Longitudinal Study for biomarkers of aging.

Sex

The scientific aspect of the caloric-restriction study in primates has been additionally confused by another political issue: sex. The original proposal for the study used only male rhesus monkeys. Scientists often prefer to use males in life-span studies; males are considered to be more "generic" biological systems, because they do not experience the dramatic hormonal changes of menopause, yet usually live as long, if not longer, than females. Already well into the study, administrators realized that the agency might be subject to criticism by feminist organizations for not including female rhesus monkeys. The scientists pointed out that it was technically unnecessary because: (1) if caloric restriction worked in males, it would work in females; (2) menopause would introduce an unproductive variable; and (3) to include both sexes would double the cost and prolong the completion date of the experiment.

Paying the Piper

To paraphrase an old proverb, whoever pays the scientists directs the science. The rhesus monkey experiment is funded by the National Institute on Aging, a division of the National Institutes of Health, an agency of the Department of Health and Human Services, of the United States federal government. Not surprisingly, female rhesus monkeys are now a part of the study. Thus, the data from this research may be scientifically irrelevant but will be politically correct.

THE BENEFITS OF CALORIC RESTRICTION

The beginnings of modern science can be attributed to folk medicine. The use of caloric restriction is particularly indebted to such a heritage. Sobriety and moderation in all things are time-honored principles of human life. The validity of these principles in relation to diet has long been recognized.

A well-documented regimen of caloric restriction comes from Luigi Cornaro, a Venetian nobleman who reportedly lived from 1464 to 1565, slightly over one hundred years. By the time he was forty, Cornaro was virtually on his deathbed from debauchery. He was told by his physicians that either he adopt a strict lifestyle of sobriety in all things, mostly eating and drinking, or he would be dead within a few months.

Cornaro became a fanatic about his regimen, subsisting on a daily diet of no more than twelve ounces of solid food and fourteen ounces of wine. He claims he was never ill again, except once when he gave up the diet. Throughout his long lifetime he was notably productive. He was active in architecture and civic affairs. He constructed four villas, and wrote books and articles on many subjects. At the age of eighty-three, he outlined his dietary regimen for longevity in his book *Discorsi della vita sobria* (*Discourse on the Sober Life*), which he rewrote three times by the time he was ninety-five. Luigi Cornaro is one early exemplar of caloric restriction as a life-extension technique.

CALORIC-RESTRICTION RESEARCH IN THE 20TH CENTURY

The modern history of caloric restriction and its relationship to life extension began in the early 1900s. Moreschi in 1903 and Rouse in 1914 each investigated the effects of a restricted diet on the incidence of tumors. They noticed that in the calorically restricted group not only was the number of tumors greatly reduced, but the overall survival rate greatly increased. In 1935, Clive McCay conducted a definitive caloric-restriction experiment.

In this particular experiment, about 40 percent of the rats' food was protein, 10 percent lard, 10 percent sugar, and 22 percent starch. The remainder was oil, fiber, vitamins, and minerals. Ironically, this diet would be fairly close to a low-fat, well-balanced, "junk food" diet of contemporary standards. The control animals were allowed to eat all they wanted. For the experimental group, food was withdrawn periodically so that their body weights were maintained at approximately their juvenile weight. Subsequently, the calorically restricted animals weighed about 40 percent less than the unrestricted ones. This is important to remember because proponents of caloric restriction recommend human body weight be about what it was at the age of twenty.

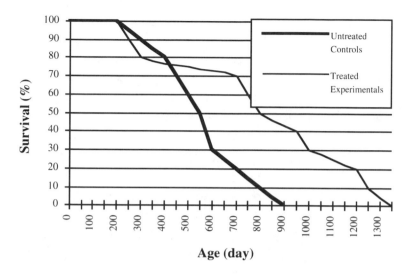

Figure 3.1 Survival Curve of Clive McCay's Original Caloric-Restriction Experiment in White Rats

Data from this chart adapted by Chadd Everone from *Life-Extension Manual.*

LIFE SPAN OF 140 YEARS

As McKay's graph shows, the average life expectancy (i.e., the point at which 50 percent of the group is still surviving) was increased from 550 days in the controls to 800 days in the calorically restricted group! That represents an increase of about 60 percent. The maximum life span was increased from 950 days in the controls to 1,350 days in the restricted group, which represents an increase of about 42 percent. If the same effect were to hold true for humans, the average life expectancy would be increased from 70 years to about 112 years, and the maximum life span would be increased from about 100 to 140 years!

In a subsequent experiment by S. Leto and other investigators, comparable life extension was achieved with the nutrient ratios changed to 26 percent protein, 4 percent lard, 49 percent sugar, and 15 percent starch, plus vitamins and minerals. In other words, about one-half of the calories in this experiment came from sugar. No doubt this will come as welcome news to many who might be of that particular persuasion!

Since McCay's first experiment in 1935, life extension via caloric restriction has been reproduced over a hundred times in many species. As long as caloric restriction is kept to about 30 to 40 percent of what is normally eaten, and vitamins and minerals are included, there has been no evidence of detrimental effect. Indeed, it can be said that because the maximum genetic life span has been increased, there is, by definition, no detrimental effect.

Life extension achieved by caloric restriction seems to be gained by slowing the fundamental aging process or processes. This maintains biological vitality and prevents or postpones disease, and the person will feel better and be healthier. After caloric restriction becomes a regular routine, appetite naturally abates and deprivation is not an issue.

Of course, the practice of caloric restriction should be avoided during pregnancy because of possible complications in fetal development, and during lactation due to increased caloric needs to supply food for two. Also, this method should be avoided during childhood because it causes delayed maturation of most systems.

ROY WALFORD: ONE SCIENTIST IN PARTICULAR

Since McCay, there have been hundreds of researchers who have contributed to the science of caloric restriction. One of the leading investigators has been Roy Walford, M.D., a professor in the Department of Pathology, School of Medicine, University of California at Los Angeles. Tracking his career will give a good understanding into the general progression of events, both in gerontology and in life extension.

In 1966, historian Gerald Gruman classified life-extensionists into three main philosophical camps: "meliorists," "incrementalists," and "immortalists." The meliorists are of the belief that the condition of the aged can be made better, more comfortable, less disease prone, more productive and happier, but that life extension per se either cannot or should not be attempted. Most gerontologists are still of this orientation with the majority of public resources going into the psychology and sociology of aging and into geriatric medicine. Incrementalists believe that emphasis should be given to developing methods to incrementally increase the life span, which consequently will have the effect of ameliorating the condition of the aged and will give additional time to work on further means toward longevity. Immortalists believe that most of the effort should be focused on understanding the fundamental causes of aging so that methods can be developed for solving the problem altogether, and eventually the development of non-aging human beings can be achieved.

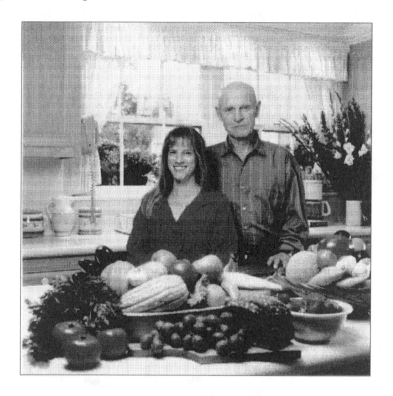

Figure 3.2 Roy Walford With His Daughter Lisa
Photo courtesy of Four Walls Eight Windows.

Roy Walford has always been overtly an incrementalist and semi-covertly an immortalist. He was originally trained as a medical doctor. This training may explain his impulse to actually solve a problem rather than, like many researchers, simply analyze and theorize about it. Instead of taking on a routine practice, Walford pursued research medicine. Early on he specialized in the immune system. Since the 1950s, he has investigated numerous aspects of immunity and published several hundred scientific reports, individually and with other investigators.

Walford is recognized as a relatively conservative scientist with a reputation for making significant contributions. In addition to his teaching, laboratory work, and publishing, he has done field work in the Amazon jungle, studying the immunology of the Tukuna Indians. He was the physician and medical researcher for the Biosphere 2 in Oracle, Arizona. Biosphere 2 was a major experiment in the early 1990s that involved humans living in a closed-cycle ecological system for several years. It served as a model for space colonization and sustainable Earth systems. From the Amazon, to the Space Station, and back to the laboratory to study life extension—Roy Walford is an intriguing and dynamic personality.

YOUTHFULNESS AND LONGEVITY

Mice on these [calorically restricted] regimens display anatomic and certain immune functional changes which suggest that the immune system may mature less rapidly and stay 'younger' longer than in the controls. Furthermore, dietary restriction results in prolongation of life span.

—Roy Walford
"Immune Function and Survival in a Long-Lived
Mouse Strain Subjected to Undernutrition"
Gerontologia

Early in his career, Walford became interested in autoimmune reaction, an immune reaction to one's self, as a significant cause of aging. In 1969, he authored one of the first books in this area titled *The Immunologic Theory of Aging*. During this early stage, Walford pursued straightforward gerontology. In other words, he attempted to analyze which aspects of the immune system decline with time and are directly associated with the aging process. Also in his early career, Walford pursued the idea of maximum life span as a parameter to evaluate biological phenomena. Around 1974, he started to take an interest in how the immune system functions within a situation of life-span extension. Because life extension has been enabled by caloric restriction, he became involved in that area of research.

Walford's interest grew in the idea of using the life-extension model for determining which biological systems are critical to aging. The idea is that the maximum genetic life span must have been extended by retarding the aging process. Therefore by monitoring biological systems during a caloric-restriction experiment, it can be determined which systems are critical to aging. Those systems that continue to decline along their normal trajectory are not critical. Those systems that do not decline along their normal trajectory are probably the ones responsible for the life extension.

In 1986, along with R. Weindruch, Walford reported the following caloric-restriction study:

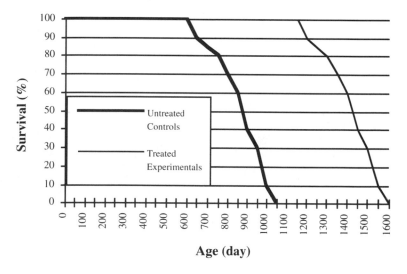

Figure 3.3 Survival Curve of Caloric Restriction in Mice
(R. Weindruch, Roy Walford)

Compare this data with the previous graph of McCay's experiment in 1935. The percentage increase in average life expectancy and maximum life span are quite similar.

From his research in caloric restriction and immunology, in 1986 Walford wrote *The 120-Year Diet: How to Double Your Vital Years*, where he reviews the scientific work. He makes the case that it will work in humans and prescribes a restricted diet that he uses himself. A leading nutritionist wrote a critical review of the book, stating that the idea of 120 years of life was outrageous. Walford's reputation as a scientist was so conservative that the reviewer speculated the book's title was forced on him by the publisher for advertising purposes. But Walford immediately published a rebuttal in an editorial letter. He rebuked the critic politely but curtly, saying that the reviewer obviously had not read the book. If he had he would have known that 120 years was precisely and literally what Walford meant.

Caloric restriction slows aging and extends the maximum life span. This has been proven by research from Walford and other scientists. The focus is now on what caloric restriction tells us about the underlying mechanisms of aging itself. In other words, what biological systems are affected by caloric restriction so as to cause life extension? Some of the main findings can be summarized as follows.

SYSTEMS AFFECTED BY CALORIC RESTRICTION

Caloric restriction maintains the protein synthesis of cells in general by means of preserving the number of receptors for insulin-like growth factor-1 thereby enabling the bio-availability of growth hormone. One of the manifestations of this is to keep the level of serum glucose from increasing, as it does normally in aging. A higher level of glucose denatures proteins and is an aging mechanism. One sees this in diabetes, which is a model of accelerated aging.

Oxidative damage to DNA appears to be a major contributor to cancer and aging. Caloric restriction lowers oxidative damage due to by-products of metabolism.

Caloric restriction reduces metabolic rate. The presence of interleukin-6 in the body is a major contributor to inflammatory responses. For example, the level of cytokine in the body increases with aging. Interleukin-6 is believed to be the cause of several diseases that are common in later life including lymphoma, osteoporosis, and Alzheimer's disease. The age-associated increase in the body's production of interleukin-6 is significantly reduced by caloric restriction. Caloric restriction delays or prevents most age-associated diseases.

Caloric restriction inhibits autoimmunity and the development of autoimmune diseases. Yet, caloric restriction maintains many immunological functions.

Caloric restriction maintains antioxidant enzymes in the liver that normally decline with age. These include manganese-superoxide dismutase, CuZn-superoxide dismutase, and glutathione peroxidase. And, caloric restriction retards the aging of the pineal gland including levels of N-acetyltransferase (NAT) activity and the levels of melatonin.

Caloric restriction results in decreased secretion of hypothalamic, pituitary, and the respective target gland hormones. The decline in hormone secretion leads to a reduction in most body functions, lowers whole body metabolism, and reduces gene expression. It thereby results in a decreased rate of aging of body tissues and longer life. These favorable effects on aging are due to caloric restriction reducing hormone secretion.

Caloric restriction slows severe neuron loss in the auditory ganglion associated with inherited deafness. This implies that caloric restriction delays the onset of genetically programmed degeneration of the nervous system.

From the research on caloric restriction, an emerging opinion among many scientists is that this method yields an extension of maximum life span by slowing the metabolic rate and thereby slowing the free-radical reactions due to metabolic by-products that cause damage to nonrenewable biological structures. Before we explore the free-radical theory of aging in more depth (in Chapter Five), we will take a look at the gerontological approach to solving the problem of aging.

CHAPTER FOUR

THEORIES OF AGING—
THE GERONTOLOGICAL
APPROACH

There are different ways to approach a solution to the problem of aging. One method is to study the aging process on a cellular plane; another is to study life-extension models. The preceding chapter focused on the life-extension model of aging as a primary point of reference; so, the viewpoint of this chapter is devoted to solving the problem of aging on a genomic, or cellular level—the approach many gerontologists use.

Imagine a perfect environment: a nutrient-dense, low-calorie diet; no exposure to radiation, infectious agents, or other toxic substances; perfectly adjusted physical exercise; minimal emotional stress; a positive attitude; the absolutely true religion; a harmonious society; and a life-support system in complete ecological balance. Within this environment your body would still age, deteriorate with time, eventually get many of the chronic diseases, and die of senescence. This naturally inevitable process would just play out over a longer time. This would not be much of an improvement unless, while you were gaining this additional time, you devoted some of your effort to correcting the entire problem of aging and deterioration at its most basic level—at the level of the genome—i.e., genetics.

THE RESILIENCE OF A CHILD

If we kept throughout life the same resistance to stress, injury, and disease that we had at the age of ten, about one half of us here today might expect to survive in seven hundred years' time.

—Alex Comfort

Evolving from the research in radiation chemistry that began in the 1950s, scientists have been able to tag cells with radioactive materials so that various cellular cycles could be observed. Scientists discovered that our human bodies are constructed of different types of cells, including *mitotic* or dividing cells, *postmitotic* or nondividing cells, and *resting* cells. Resting cells are currently not dividing but are capable of doing so under some circumstances. For example, the epithelium of the small intestine divides continuously (mitotic); brain cells are normally incapable of dividing (postmitotic); and liver and kidney cells usually do not divide but can, if enough of them are damaged (resting).

The entire body, with its trillions of different cells, originated from one cell. This cell had within it all of the information and a genetic "program" (DNA) to go about dividing into differentiated cell types. These different cell types form all of the tissues integrated into the very complex, highly adaptive system that becomes a human body. All of the information to construct the body is within molecular genetics. Personal intelligence and conscious knowledge had nothing to do with it. That is the power of DNA.

All of the information that is necessary to create you is in the genetic material of virtually every cell of your body. You could theoretically take the nucleus from one of your cells, place it into an ovum which has had its nucleus removed, stimulate that ovum to start dividing, transplant that ovum into a uterus, and in nine months a genetic copy of you would be born as an infant. This copy would go through the physical development sequence that you did. This "cloning" has been done in many kinds of life-forms, including mice. Some believe that human cloning has already been done in secret.

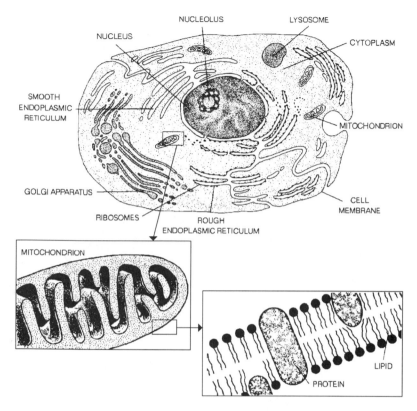

Figure 4.1 Schematic of a Typical Human Cell

Organelles are not drawn to exact scale here, to allow characteristic features to be illustrated. The membrane is a basic feature of every organelle in the cell. The location of the outer membrane of a mitochondrion is shown in this sequence of blowups; the picture would be similar for any of the other organelles or the cell membrane. Variations in composition exist, but the double lipid layer is a common feature. The heads (dark spot) of the lipid molecules have a high attraction for water and face outward; the tails (zigzag line) of the lipid molecules, which prefer an oily environment, face each other. This creates an oily layer inside the membrane. The tails of these lipid molecules are the target of lipid peroxidation, especially if the lipids are polyunsaturated. Vitamin E normally works inside the membrane to prevent peroxidation, but if the lipid is unprotected, free radicals and oxygen can cause a chain reaction which polymerizes (ties together) these lipids and disrupts the membrane. This would then impair the function of the organelle and possibly damage the cell (as a broken lysosome would, for example).

From *Secrets of Life Extension* by John Mann. Used by permission

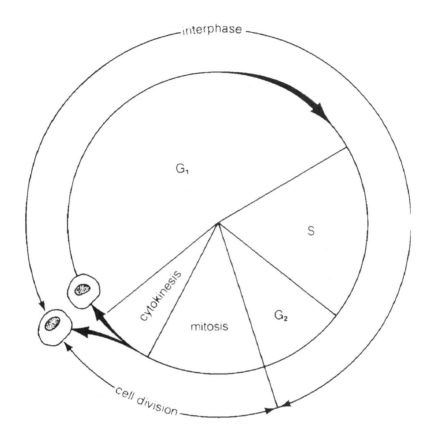

Figure 4.2 The Cell Cycle

The cell cycle. The G_1 period of interphase may be of variable length, but for a given cell type the remaining S_1, G_2 and division segments of the cycle are usually of uniform duration.

From *Introduction to Cell Biology* by Stephen L. Wolfe. Used by permission.

When a cell divides properly it reconstructs itself completely. When an aged cell, which has a lot of structural wear and tear (protein degradation) and a lot of accumulated waste (lipofuscin), goes through mitosis (cell division), two new daughter cells are created. They are capable of operating as well as the original cell.

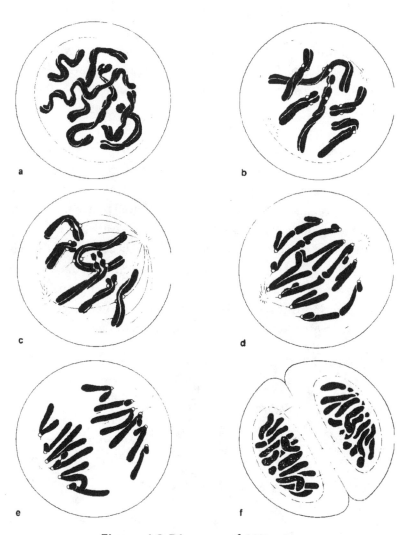

Figure 4.3 Diagram of Mitosis

From *Introduction to Cell Biology* by Stephen L. Wolfe. Used by permission.

   Nondividing, postmitotic cells, such as those in the brain, inevitably deteriorate over time. When they terminate, there is usually no replacement. All of the genetic information to redivide and recreate is in the postmitotic cell, but somehow is being inhibited from switching on when needed.

HOW THE BRAIN GROWS AND CHANGES

The neurons in the brain are called postmitotic cells, because they don't multiply after the brain structure is originally created. According to aging researcher Albert Rosenfeld, once such cells die, they are 'dead and gone forever.' However, there is some recent evidence that, under the right conditions, the brain can, in fact, grow new cells. In other words, over time, the brain gradually loses nerve cells with their synaptic connections, because of normal wear and tear, accidental injury, aging, or strokes. The actual extent and effect of brain-cell loss are in dispute. Researchers once believed that in the normal course of aging as many as 100,000 brain cells were lost every day after age thirty-five. Although it is generally believed that there is brain-cell loss over time, this high figure has been challenged by Alex Comfort, one of the world's leading gerontologists. Enthusiasts for smart drugs and nutrients assert that aging due to nerve-cell loss can be slowed by the use of brain boosters, nutrients, and drugs....

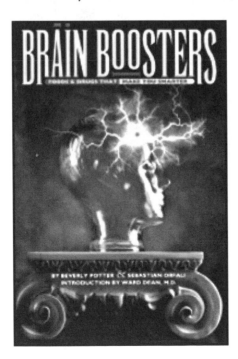

New research indicates that brain cells or neurons may change in response to experience...that the dendrites can grow new protrusions in minutes in response to new experiences. ... Thus, as you learn and have new experiences, the very structure of your brain actually changes.

—Beverly Potter, Ph.D. & Sebastian Orfali

Brain Boosters: Foods and Drugs That Make You Smarter

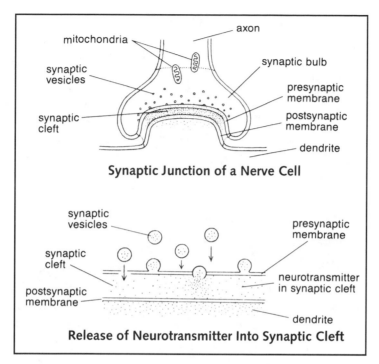

Synaptic Junction of a Nerve Cell

Release of Neurotransmitter Into Synaptic Cleft

From *Mind Food & Smart Pills: A Sourcebook for the Vitamins, Herbs, & Drugs That Can Increase Intelligence, Improve Memory, & Prevent Brain Aging* by Ross Pelton. Copyright © 1989 by Montrose P. Pelton. Used by Permission of Doubleday, a division of Bantam Doubleday Dell Publishing Group, Inc.

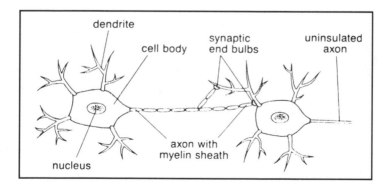

Figure 4.4 SYNAPTIC JUNCTION: Structure of Nerve Cells

From *Mind Food & Smart Pills: A Sourcebook for the Vitamins, Herbs, & Drugs That Can Increase Intelligence, Improve Memory, & Prevent Brain Aging* by Ross Pelton. Copyright © 1989 by Montrose P. Pelton. Used by Permission of Doubleday, a division of Bantam Doubleday Dell Publishing Group, Inc.

QUEST FOR CELL IMMORTALITY

Since the origin of the idea that the cell is the essential living unit, one of the important questions in biology has been whether the cell has, inherently, a definite life span or an indefinite life span. The key issue centers around the term "inherently." One experimental model for addressing this question is to study cells *in vitro*, which means living in a test-tube culture, independently of interaction with or dependence on other cells in a body.

INCREASING THE DURATION OF YOUTH

Longevity is only desirable if it increases the duration of youth, and not that of old age. The lengthening of the senescent period would be a calamity.

—Alexis Carrel
Man the Unknown

Alexis Carrel, a famous scientist in the history of physiology, initiated a study growing fibroblast cells *in vitro* from the heart of a chicken embryo. He reported in 1912 that these cells lived indefinitely. In his experiment, the cells were raised on culture plates in an incubator. They were sustained nutritionally by a crude extract from other chicken embryos. His cultured cells would divide and multiply. He would cull down the number, let them regrow, recull them, let them regrow, and so on. For over thirty years, the same batch of cells was sustained throughout thousands of cycles. In 1946, two years after Carrel's death, the experiment was abandoned.

From 1946 until the 1960s, the reigning dogma in biology was that cells had, intrinsically, a potential for infinite survival. The reason for the observed limited life span in living organisms must be due to some factor in the normal cellular milieu. There seemed to be two possibilities: (1) cells, once liberated from the body, were no longer constrained by some inhibitory factor that existed in the whole organism; or (2) some essential life-sustaining, growth factor was contained in the embryonic extract that was being fed to the cells, and this factor was lost in mature adults.

Carrel's experiment oriented gerontology and general physiology in a certain direction. On the one hand, if the life-sustaining growth factor could be isolated, it could be synthesized and delivered as a therapy to cure aging. This notion was probably the origin of what is called "cell therapy" devised around that time by Paul Niehans, a Swiss surgeon. Niehans took fresh cells from the organs of animal fetuses and injected this preparation into patients. The procedure is still used today in some clinics in Switzerland and the Bahamas. Claims of efficacy are made but most gerontologists do not take them seriously. Niehans himself aged and died at an unexceptional life span of eighty-nine years.

On the other hand was the possibility that cell mortality could be caused by some factor in the body's milieu. If so, this factor might be isolated and chemical methods found for intervention. This is probably the underlying notion for what came to be known as the "death hormone" theory. This theory, espoused by Denckla in the 1970s, subsequently appears to have been abandoned as no proof has been established.

CELLS ARE NOT INTRINSICALLY IMMORTAL

In 1961, Leonard Hayflick and Paul Moorhead overturned the "Carrellian" dogma of the natural immortality of cells. They meticulously attempted to repeat Carrel's experiment. They found that normal, cultured, embryonic fibroblasts will only divide approximately fifty times before they cease replication, deteriorate, and die. In other words, cells are not intrinsically immortal. Apparently, Carrel had been accidentally injecting new embryonic cells into his feeding medium and thereby refreshing the colony intermittently. It appeared as though the original colony was sustaining itself but, in fact, it was not. Because of Carrel's strong reputation in science and his considerable influence in the politics of science, no one challenged the veracity of his work until Hayflick and Moorhead proved otherwise in the 1960s.

In addition to demonstrating that normal cells in culture cannot divide indefinitely, Hayflick and Moorhead proposed that the intrinsic limitation on the number of times that a cell can divide might be one of the basic mechanisms of aging. This line of inquiry is still at the center of gerontological research today. But the story is not that simple.

RESETTING THE BIOLOGICAL CLOCK

Such reshuffling of genetic information when egg and sperm cells are produced or fused could perhaps serve to reprogram or reset the cell's biological clock. By this mechanism, even if the individual members of a species were programmed to die, the species would live. A human being, then, would be the germ cell's way of making more immortal germ cells.

—Leonard Hayflick
"The Serial Cultivation of Human Diploid Cell Strains"
Experimental Cell Research

CELL DIVISION IS AT THE HEART OF THE MATTER

There are some strange twists to the phenomena of cell division. Normal cells are not intrinsically immortal—that fact is well established. Cancer cells, however, seem to be immortal *in vitro*. Cancer cells are normal cells that have differentiated and reverted to an unregulated, rapidly dividing state. As long as a cancer cell can feed, it appears to keep multiplying and live forever. The famous HeLa cells, for example, are cancer cells taken from the cervix of a woman in 1952 by George O. Gey at Johns Hopkins University School of Medicine. These cells have been propagated and sent all over the world for study and are still multiplying to this day.

Normal differentiated cells have the capacity to divide and regenerate themselves only a finite number of times (50 +/− 10 times). This is known as the "Hayflick phenomenon." But the same cells, if genetically transformed into cancer seem to have the ability to divide and regenerate themselves forever.

The relevance of the Hayflick phenomenon to the normal process of aging has always been subject to question. The basis of the criticism is quite simple: Cells living in culture are in a completely different situation from cells living in a body. Their behavior in culture may not be a proper model to study any normal biological processes, including aging. Objections to this model have been reviewed extensively by J. A. Witkowski in an article titled "Cell Aging *in Vitro*—An Historical Perspective."

Further, researcher Charles Daniel has performed experiments involving the serial transplantation of mouse mammary glands, demonstrating that the same tissue can survive for more than four full life spans. If there is a Hayflick limit in living systems, it is probably not a limiting factor within the normal life span of a whole organism. Daniel does, however, consider the limitation of cell replication to be a fundamental mechanism in aging and Witkowski holds the discovery of cell aging in culture to be a "scientific revolution." Irrespective of the precise applicability of the Hayflick phenomenon to aging, cell division probably lies at the heart of the matter.

REJUVENATION AND CELL PROLIFERATION

While caloric restriction definitely slows aging and can increase a healthy life span, it does not stop aging. More importantly, it does not reverse aging. To reverse aging may require the controlled induction of *eumitosis*. In other words, full biological regeneration does occur naturally when a cell divides properly.

Caloric restriction retards the cell's rate of operation to preserve it longer. Antioxidants counter free radicals and other degradative processes within the cells. The administration of growth hormone, or dehydroepiandrosterone (DHEA), supplements hormones that have declined. There are many other ways people might conceive to reconstruct the damage to the cell that occurs from normal wear and tear or disease. Theoretically, a more direct approach would be to figure out how to signal the cell to redivide properly when needed. The cell already contains this information. If we could figure out how to initiate the process, the genetic and cytoplasmic systems would do the detail work.

"The proliferation theory of rejuvenation" is a term invented by David Danner of the Laboratory of Molecular Genetics at the National Institute on Aging. In his paper, he describes his perspective as follows.

PROLIFERATION THEORY OF REJUVENATION

This theory assumes that aging is due to the accumulation of multiple forms of molecular damage and that rejuvenation is due to repair. . .it is proposed that cell proliferation is required for full rejuvenation.

—David Danner
Paper presented to the National Institute on Aging

By cell proliferation Danner means the induction of eumitosis or proper division. Cell proliferation is an extremely active area of science. Over twenty thousand original citations on this topic were deposited in the Medline data bank in the early 1990s—a tremendous number of reports. The intensity of focus of this research can be attributed to progress in cell culture techniques and new instruments such as molecular probes. These advances make it possible to study the details of the cell cycle. Cell proliferation is of interest not only to aging research, but is essential to understanding cancer and all aspects of medicine. This is a profound convergence that could represent a major leap forward in medicine.

CELL SENESCENCE

The area of cell senescence and regeneration is new and the data is so far disparate. There is a maze of technicalities that have not been substantiated. Cell senescence occurs for the following reasons: random accumulation of cellular damage that is not repaired, errors in synthesis, and DNA damage; and a genetic program that is associated with causing the cell to become differentiated. The loss of the cell's ability to proliferate is an active process. This process is a blocking of the reinitiation of DNA synthesis that causes mitosis or cell division. The reinitiation of controlled cell division depends on signals from stimulatory and inhibitory growth factors and on the genes or gene products that interact with these factors. Reproductive failure, the inability of controlled eumitosis and cell proliferation, is the fundamental characteristic of cellular senescence. Research on the molecular basis of cell senescence and aging is definitely an area to keep an eye on.

TRANSFORMATION

The human body dies only because we have forgotten how to transform it and change it.

—Antonin Artaud
Theater and Science

THE IMPORTANCE OF HOST VITALITY

As Louis Pasteur recognized in the later part of the 1800s, the fundamental cause of disease is not external pathogens but rather host vitality. Host vitality is the general health and immune strength of the organism. Over the last hundred years, medicine, public sanitation, personal hygiene, and industrialization have made considerable gains

on major external pathogens. That approach to health care is important, but can only go so far. The amount of resources required to get a
benefit in terms of life extension has almost reached the point of
diminishing returns. In order to sustain progress, one place for medical
research is a deeper level of biological control. That may be the
manipulation of cells to replicate themselves properly—in other words,
cell regeneration. Thus, the future of medicine and the pursuit of life
extension go hand in hand.

CHAPTER FIVE

THE FREE-RADICAL THEORY OF AGING

The free-radical theory of aging targets what is widely believed to be the most immediate cause of aging. What are free radicals? A free radical is a portion of a molecule that either has one extra electron, or is missing an electron. Because of this imbalance, free radicals are unstable and usually very reactive, and will attempt to bond with almost any other molecule they bump into. The process of normal metabolism generates these free radicals, which can damage tissue through oxidative chain reactions and cross-linkage. Cells naturally have defense systems that generate antioxidants; but inevitably damage occurs. Because free radicals are generated in every cell type, all biological systems are affected. This chapter takes a look at the affect that free radicals have on the mechanism of aging.

The aspect of metabolism relevant to life extension involves the mitochondrion. The mitochondrion utilizes oxygen and water and a simplified sugar called pyruvate to synthesize adenosine triphosphate (ATP). ATP is an energy molecule that enables the body to produce its polymers—vitamins, proteins, hormones, and enzymes. In the process of this energy conversion and synthesis of polymers, normal chemical by-products are constantly generated called "free radicals."

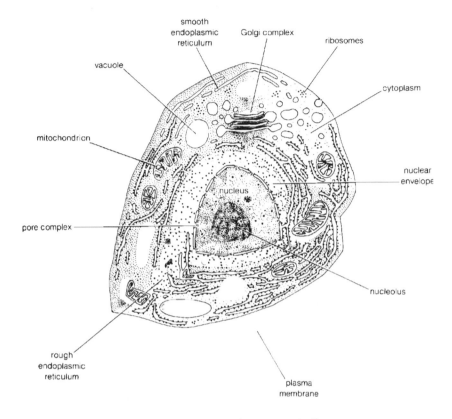

Figure 5.1 A Eukaryotic Cell

Structures typically seen in electron micrographs of eukaryotic cells.

From *Introduction to Cell Biology* by Stephen L. Wolfe. Used by Permission.

PREMATURE DEATH

Very few individuals, if any, reach their potential maximum
life span; they die instead prematurely of a wide variety of diseases—the vast majority being free-radical diseases.

—Denham Harman, M.D., Ph.D.

FREE RADICALS

Besides being an everyday chemical by-product, free radicals can also be created due to external factors. Free radicals can be formed by exposure to radiation, pollution, pesticides, dietary substances, and even from the air we breathe or from toxic residues created by stress or exhaustion. For example, exposure to passive smoke from cigarettes sets loose *billions* of free radicals into the blood stream. Twentieth-century lifestyles in combination with the toxic-filled environment contribute to an overabundance of free-radical production. Antioxidants are molecular substances that can inactivate free radicals. The human body's natural ability to produce antioxidants has not evolved quickly enough to deal with today's excessive amounts of externally caused free-radical production. Thus, degenerative diseases are rampant.

FREE-RADICAL DAMAGE

Unfortunately, the molecule that loses its electron to a free radical is damaged and may even be destroyed. It's like the married man who loses his wife to another man, and is rendered nonfunctional by the depression that results.

As attacks by free radicals increase over time with aging, more healthy molecules are damaged and destroyed. This contributes to the chronic degenerative diseases and decline in brain power. In fact, free radicals can create chain reactions of ever-increasing damage, because when a free radical steals an electron from another molecule, this produces another free radical, which goes on to seek out another molecule to steal from. So there's a kind of domino effect that contributes to further disrupting bodily and brain functioning on the cellular level.

—Beverly Potter, Ph.D. and Sebastian Orfali
Brain Boosters: Foods & Drugs That Make You Smarter

When free radicals run rampant, they promiscuously bond with almost anything, including proteins, other polymer molecules such as hormones and enzymes, and even with DNA. This reaction can cause different effects, which include cross-linkage and chain scission. In chain scission, the polymers that react with the free radical are cut into small pieces and their structure turns putty-like. In cross-linkage, the polymers that react with the free radical are bound together. If this binding is excessive, the substance becomes brittle and inelastic.

Both chain scission and cross-linkage occur in metabolic processes. In the study of aging, however, cross-linkage has received most of the attention.

CROSS-LINKAGE

Here are two examples to illustrate cross-linkage. Rubber, when it comes originally from the sap of trees, is a viscous liquid. The polymers are cross-linked only to the point of biological viability for the rubber plant. To make rubber useful it must be toughened enough to make it elastic but not brittle. By treating the rubber with heat and chemicals, its polymers become appropriately cross-linked. If the rubber is over-treated, however, or if it is exposed for a long time to oxygen or ultraviolet radiation, the cross-linkage of the polymers progresses to the point of excess and the rubber disintegrates.

Another example of cross-linkage happens when an egg is cooked. Before the egg is heated, its protein is transparent, gelatinous, and somewhat tough to the touch. After the egg is heated, however, the protein becomes massively cross-linked–light can no longer pass through the protein, but it is reflected from it; and the protein crumbles easily.

To control cross-linkage, all living organisms manufacture anti-oxidants or obtain them in food.

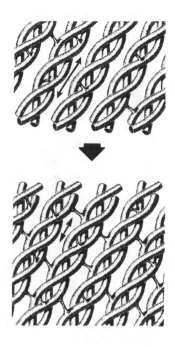

Figure 5.2 Collagen and Cross-Linking of Collagen

This model of collagen shows the remarkable architecture of connective tissue. Each of the tube structures represents a chain of amino acids. Three such chains twisted together in a spiral (a triple helix) are considered a unit of collagen. Many of these units are joined end-to-end to form long, continuous threads. In turn, these continuous threads are stacked side by side to form larger strands. A small section of one of those strands is shown here.

During youth, there is a moderate amount of cross-linking to tie the collagen threads to each other (shown in the top half of the picture). As a result, the collagen threads slide past each other, and the connective tissue is quite elastic. With increasing age, more cross-links are formed; these tie more collagen threads to each other, and the sliding of threads past each other becomes greatly restricted (shown in the bottom half of this picture). The result is less-elastic connective tissue.

From *Secrets of Life Extension* by John Mann. Used by permission.

NATURAL MECHANISMS FOR HANDLING FREE RADICALS

Aerobic organisms have evolved complex mechanisms to prevent uncontrolled free-radical production and oxidative damage. In mammals, these include the cytochrome oxidases, reduced glutathione, glutathione peroxidase and reductase, superoxide dismutase and catalase. Glutathione functions to protect protein sulfhydryl groups by serving as a substrate for selenium dependent glutathione peroxidase, the enzyme that removes hydrogen peroxides and thus protects membrane lipids from auto-oxidation. In addition, glutathione acts as a natural intracellular antioxidant protecting many enzymes that require the presence of free sulfhydryl groups and are inactivated or inhibited if these groups are oxidized. Glutathione also acts to detoxify halogenated aliphatic and aromatic hydrocarbons. Glutathione is kept in its reduced, active form by the enzyme, glutathione reductase. Glutathione is made up of cysteine, glycine, and glutamic acid.

Superoxide dismutase is an enzyme found generally in aerobic cells and is responsible for conversion of superoxide radical to hydrogen peroxide and molecular oxygen. It exists in two forms—the mitochondrial form being manganese-dependent, and the cytosol form containing copper and zinc. The enzyme catalase then converts hydrogen peroxide to nonreactive oxygen and water. The cytochromes act as electron-transferring proteins in the respiratory chain and thus are important mediators in the reduction of oxygen and the prevention of formation of free radicals. Ubiquinone is an electron-carrying coenzyme that also participates in this transfer of electrons. The proper functioning of the electron transport chain also depends upon the niacin and riboflavin-dependent coenzymes NAD+, NADP+, FMN, and FAD.

—Karuna Corp.—Technical Sheet
Professional Information Series
Free Radicals and Antioxidant Coping Mechanisms

In industrial chemistry, synthesized antioxidants can be added to materials to retard deterioration. Antioxidants are also used as a common food additive to retain "freshness."

DENHAM HARMAN'S DECADES OF RESEARCH

In 1956, Dr. Denham Harman presented his original proposal that free-radical reactions and the resulting cross-linkage might be a significant factor in biological aging, and that life span could be expanded by adding antioxidants to the diet. Since that time, numerous investigators have contributed to research in this area. Over the years, Harman himself has continued to keep pace with developments.

LIVING LONGER, BETTER

The basic purpose of all this business is: How do we get to live longer better? If we can't live longer, let's live better. I think we can do both, though.

—Denham Harman
quoted in *The Youth Doctors*
Patrick McGrady, Jr.

EFFECTS OF RADIATION

Ionizing radiation damages cells in two ways. Low levels of radiation cause cells to generate free radicals; free-radical damage can lead to excessive cross-linkage and cell destruction. High levels of radiation damage DNA and either cause cells to mutate or to lose the ability to divide. Consequently, the cells die. From animal studies as well as human exposures, it has been documented that radiation causes cancers, shortens life span, and ostensibly accelerates aging. It has also been documented that antioxidants can counteract the effects of radiation!

CAN ANTIOXIDANTS SLOW AGING & EXTEND LIFE?

The following hypothesis arose: Radiation causes accelerated aging by inducing excessive free-radical reactions. These free-radical reactions can be inhibited by the administration of antioxidants. Similarly, normal human aging might be caused, over a long period of time, by low-level, free-radical reactions generated by normal cell metabolism and environmental stresses. Therefore, the ingestion of antioxidants should slow aging and thereby extend the human life span.

Whether antioxidants slow aging and extend life span needs to be explored more fully. Such claims are being made, and many people are taking antioxidants for life-extension purposes, as well as for health and general well-being.

Harman's initial experiments in antioxidant administration were encouraging. Subsequent research by other investigators, however, has produced a plethora of variable results. There are ambiguities within the free-radical theory of aging.

One of the synthetic antioxidants, butylated hydroxytoluene (BHT), caused an early death at the intended therapeutic level. The antioxidants ethoxyquin and 2-mercaptoethylamine (both synthetic) have also been shown to produce a shortened life span in mice. But factors other than the antioxidants themselves may be responsible for disparity in data. Hypotheses and conclusions vary. For example, some researchers have determined that antioxidants do not inhibit aging but can improve survival under conditions of exposure to toxins. Other researchers have reached different conclusions. Data are still ambiguous at best. What is not always accounted for is that as a matter of course almost all experimental animals have vitamins and minerals already supplemented into their feed as a normal part of their diet. A "vitamin-fortified" diet naturally includes some of the antioxidants at an acceptable level.

It has been reported that adding antioxidants can make the food taste so bad that the experimental animals undereat. They are therefore modestly restricted calorically, which has already been proven to extend the survival curve. Some investigators do not monitor the food intake or body weights of the animals as a matter of course. Thus the caloric-restriction aspect has been an ever-present, potential component in most life-extension research whether it is officially part of the experiment or not.

ANIMAL EXPERIMENTATION

Within all biological systems, the natural manufacture of a chemical is reduced if that chemical is supplemented. In 1984 Richard Cutler, a senior scientist with the National Institute on Aging, proposed that the administration of antioxidants may be ineffective in slowing aging because when antioxidants are supplemented the cells decrease production of their own intrinsic antioxidants. Cutler reasoned that supplementing antioxidants would reduce endogenous production and there would be no net increase in available antioxidants. He proposed to genetically engineer a mouse that would naturally overproduce antioxidants. He would use that mouse to test whether or not free antioxidants slow aging.

Cutler has yet to publish any findings regarding the genetically altered mouse, but a parallel experiment was performed by investigators Orr and Sohal in 1994, using a fruit fly, *Drosophila melanogaster*. They reported a 30 percent increase in maximum life span when the flies were genetically altered to over-express their production of an intrinsic antioxidant, copper-zinc superoxide dismutase and catalase. In addition, they reported a lower amount of protein oxidative damage, a delay in the loss of physical performance, and a delay of the mortality rate. All of these results reinforce the free-radical theory of aging and the role of antioxidant surveillance in life extension. The mouse, as well as the fruit fly, however, are not the best representative models for human aging— humans are.

THE ANTIOXIDANT STATUS OF AN
INDIVIDUAL IS VERY IMPORTANT

Cutler, diligently hard at work, published an article in the early 1990s titled "Antioxidants and Aging" in the *American Journal of Clinical Nutrition*. His abstract reads as follows.

ANTIOXIDANTS AND AGING

Aging in mammalian species appears to be the result of normal developmental and metabolic processes. In spite of the vast complexity of aging processes, relatively less complex processes such as longevity determinant genes may exist governing aging rate. Much experimental data exists indicating a causative role of oxyradicals in aging processes. In testing the hypothesis that antioxidants may represent longevity determinant genes, a positive correlation in the tissue concentration of specific antioxidants with life span of mammals was found. These antioxidants include superoxide dismutase, carotenoids, alpha-tocopherol, and uric acid. We also found that the resistance of tissues to spontaneous auto-oxidation and the amount of oxidative damage to DNA correlates inversely with life span of mammals. These results suggest a role of oxyradicals in causing aging and that the antioxidant status of an individual could be important in determining frequency of age-dependent diseases and duration of general health maintenance.

—Richard G. Cutler
American Journal of Clinical Nutrition

The efficacy of caloric restriction on life extension certainly seems to have been proven satisfactorily within the boundaries of laboratory research. Since our technological abilities are expanding at an exponential rate, hopefully all of the other factors that contribute to prolonging life will be known someday. Until that day comes, aspects of every possible life-extension method or device will be subject to continual experimentation and research, humans being the inquisitive mammals that they are.

PROLONGATION OF LIFE SPAN

Dietary caloric restriction is the most effective known strategy for prolongation of life span in mammals.

—R. Weindruch and R. Walford
The Retardation of Aging and Disease by Dietary Restriction

Let's review some benefits of caloric restriction. By restricting caloric intake the rate of metabolism is slowed. This makes cellular processes more efficient, reducing the generation of free radicals, and decreasing the oxidative damage that free radicals cause. Cellular structures last longer and there is a lower frequency of damage to DNA. Reducing food intake also reduces the amount of toxins the body must process. Normal food contains an immense amount of toxic substances that causes a fair portion of metabolic stress, so eating less leads to metabolic stress reduction. There is a limit to what caloric restriction can achieve because it only slows the degenerative processes of aging. It does not completely stop or reverse aging; so we do need to deal with aging on a cellular level.

What happens when the technique of caloric restriction is combined with other proposed life-extension therapies? Roy Walford and colleagues decided to do just that. They added particular antioxidants as suppleents to animals which were already on a calorically restricted diet. The data were presented in a paper titled "Dietary Restriction Alone and in Combination with Oral Ethoxyquin/2-Mercaptoethylamine in Mice" published in the *Journal of Gerontology*.

A SHORTENED LIFE SPAN

To investigate effects of dietary caloric restriction combined with antioxidant feeding, long-lived hybrid mice were divided into four dietary groups at weaning, and followed until natural death. Groups "C" and "R" received control (97kcal/wk) and restricted (56 kcal/wk) diets respectively. Groups "C + alpha ox" and "R"+ alpha ox" received C or R diets supplemented with an antioxidant mixture (2-mercaptoethylamine plus ethoxyquin). R mice (mean life span 41 months) significantly outlived the other three groups (mean life span 30–34 months). Hepatic degeneration and increased hepatoma in the R + alpha ox group suggested unusual hepatotoxicity of this regimen. Antioxidants had little effect on splenic cell mitogen response in similarly fed mice sacrificed at 12–15 months. Gompertz analysis suggests that the beneficial effect of dietary restriction may be due to reductions in initial vulnerability or rate-of-aging parameters, or both, and that the relative influence of each factor may vary with animal strain and dietary-restriction protocol used.

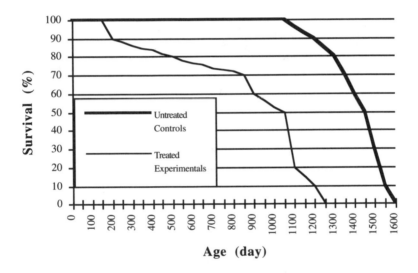

Figure 5.3 Combining Dietary Restriction and Antioxidant Supplementation

S. Harris, R. Weindruch, G. Smith, M. R. Mickey, and R. Walford, "Dietary Restriction Alone and in Combination with Oral Ethoxyquin/2–Mercaptoethylamine in Mice," *Journal of Gerontology*.

A picture tells a thousand words. Walford's graph shows that the antioxidants ethoxyquin and 2–mercaptoethylamine administered to calorically restricted animals *shortened* their life span. Compare this graph with Walford's previous caloric-restriction experiment on page 57 of Chapter Three.

In both experiments, the calorically restricted animals had greatly extended life spans—these data support the theory that caloric restriction is the important component. But the antioxidant factor is variable. The "normal" group receiving antioxidant supplements had better survival curves than the animals fed normally with no antioxidant supplementation.

The group receiving the calorically restricted regimen and also receiving antioxidants ethoxyquin and 2–mercaptoethylamine, however, had significantly *worse* survival curves than those calorically restricted and not consuming those antioxidants. Does this sound confusing? In other words, data from *these* particular experiments seem to show that if a calorically restricted diet is maintained, certain antioxidants should not be supplemented into the diet—but if a normal diet is eaten, one should consider supplementing antioxidants. But this conclusion has hidden variables. The diet of laboratory mice already includes antioxidants in many of its constituents: casein, vitamin-free test; cornstarch; dextrose; corn oil; mineral mixture; USP VIV4; fiber; vitamin mixture; brewer's yeast; zinc oxide.

The experimenters' conclusions for this particular experiment focus on the dietary-restriction component. They state that the beneficial effect of dietary restriction may be due to reductions in initial vulnerability; reductions in rate-of-aging parameters; *both* reductions in initial vulnerability and in rate-of-aging parameters; and that the relative influence of each factor may vary with animal strain and dietary-restriction protocol used. A lot of variables here! We can speculate as to other reasons why these results were obtained. Attempting to push the antioxidant mechanism beyond what caloric restriction provides might reverse the beneficial effect of caloric restriction by some unexplained mechanism.

Another reason for the results might be that those specific antioxidants consumed, ethoxyquin/2-mercaptoethylamine, are just not effective in increasing life span, although this would not discount that other antioxidants might be effective in extending the length of life.

Finally, animal husbandry methods are another factor toward the disparity in data samples. When animal husbandry methods are improved such that the control animals are living optimally, the addition of some antioxidants do not always have a beneficial effect. The confusion and contradictions seem to originate from the issue of optimal versus suboptimal conditions. When experimental and control animals are maintained poorly, their survival curves are suboptimal. If, for example, their food is rancid or their hygiene is poor, they have shortened average and maximum life spans. In such situations, when antioxidants are added to the diet of the experimentals, some disease is either prevented or delayed and the experimental group has an improved survival curve in comparison to the controls.

Emotional, spiritual, physical, and psychological factors are variable components that are difficult to account for, especially in humans, let alone laboratory animals, and are contributing factors on many tangible levels. Animals used in experiments have no choice in the matter. Their unwillingness to sacrifice their life and their inability to escape from such experimentation must affect at least their emotional state, which could affect the results of any experimentation.

Another factor is the dosage. Optimal dosage can be determined for humans, but in small animals optimal dosage is usually not the key component within the experiments. A toxicity level would be easy to reach in tiny mammals.

MORE IS NOT ALWAYS BETTER

Mammals have evolved slowly on planet Earth, with plenty of time to develop complex internal mechanisms to inhibit rampant free-radical production and oxidative damage. This century has introduced an abundance of potentially lethal substances, however, that our present rate of evolution has not prepared us for. We need a little external help.

The only external antioxidants traditionally available are from dietary plant sources. The human body never had the opportunity to consume synthetic antioxidants until supplements were chemically developed. It is relatively difficult to overdose on the amount of vitamin

A found in leafy greens, for example, but thanks to the invention of vitamin pills, the potential to overdose on little pills is possible. There is definitely a toxic level that can be reached, so it is important to take the "right dose," which varies daily for every individual. Like Goldilock's dilemma with food that was "too hot, too cold, or just right," there are also levels of "too much, too little, and just right" in the realm of supplements.

Think about what oxidation is—oxidation is how you live, how you breathe, how you function. Too much oxidation is harmful. When those rascally little free-radicals raise chaos on the cellular level anything can happen. But too *little* oxidation, which could occur if an excessive amount of antioxidants are consumed, is also damaging. Copious antioxidant ingestion can cause symptoms ranging from fatigue to liver damage. The body seeks equilibrium. There needs to be a balanced amount taken, enough so that excessive free-radical damage does not occur, and not so much that it goes the other way and the body is running on empty.

CONSUMING ANTIOXIDANTS

Nutritional supplements seem to be almost a requirement in the regimens of many health enthusiasts. It is probable that health and subsequent youthful longevity may be enhanced by the addition of nutritional supplements to the diet. This section examines supplements used to enhance quality of life and reduce free-radical damage intracel-lularly.

Many people take nutritional supplements on blind faith. Often, "how I feel" is the only criterion for whether or not these agents are doing any good. How a person "feels" is always ambiguous. It is subject to suggestion, fear, hope, and whatever else may invoke a placebo effect. A good source for guidelines for subjective self-analysis on nutritional status are provided in Dr. Richard Passwater's book *Supernutrition for Healthy Hearts.*

ANTIOXIDANTS & FREE-RADICAL DEACTIVATORS

Many life-extension experiments in laboratory animals have been done with nutrient antioxidants. Antioxidants are also among the least expensive and most accessible life-extension substances. Antioxidants apparently work by slowing down the dangerous peroxidation of lipids, usually by presenting themselves as sacrificial material to be oxidized and subsequently use up the oxygen before it can react with the lipids. The products of such reactions are relatively stable and harmless compounds, which the body has little trouble metabolizing and eliminating. Free-radical deactivators, sometimes called free-radical "scavengers," operate on a similar principle, reacting harmlessly with free radicals before these can react dangerously with vital components of the body. Most often, a substance that prevents peroxidation will also deactivate free radicals.

USE OF DIETARY SUPPLEMENTS

Auto-oxidation appears to play a key role in aging. Experiments have shown a striking increase in the longevity of laboratory animals whose diet was supplemented with antioxidants. The natural antioxidant vitamin E also seems to be important in the maintenance of cell function. There appears to be little reason to doubt that the judicious use and development of dietary supplements will add significantly to healthy life expectancy.

—Bernard Strehler
Santa Barbara Gerontology Conference

Antioxidants play different roles: as primary or secondary agents; as water-solubles or lipid-solubles; and have activity in varied sites, e.g., microsomes, mitochondria, or cell membranes. For this reason, and because these substances are mutually potentiating, an appropriate mixture seems to be the most valuable. Humans are complex biological systems—individual nutritional needs vary daily, due to exposure to environmental toxins, disease states, metabolism, radiation exposure, and consumption of carcinogenic compounds in foods. The efficacy of ideal dosages and combinations is difficult to determine. Objective means for assessing the effectiveness of nutritional supplements, their proper dosages, and how well they are being absorbed include hair analysis, essential metabolic analysis, and computerized diet analysis. Information regarding these objective tests are included in Chapter Eight.

The wisest approach to using dietary supplements is to combine moderate amounts of various supplements, rather than use large quantities of any single agent. This approach would minimize the risk of toxic or allergic reactions to any one or more of the substances to which the individual may be sensitive, or which may be toxic in large amounts. It is best to use mainly those antioxidants that are already a part of a natural diet. It can be estimated that a majority of the population, however, does not meet the USDA daily requirements for consumption of fruits (2–4 servings) and vegetables (3–5 servings). Since fruits and vegetables are the primary sources of antioxidant nutrients, yet not enough are consumed, supplementation with nutritional antioxidants may be necessary to provide essential nutrients and protection against free-radical marauders. Appropriate levels of antioxidants may also reduce the risk of cancer, cardiovascular disease, and other diseases that shorten the life span.

AN ADDITIONAL FORTY YEARS OF YOUTHFUL LIFE

Antioxidant therapy alone should add five to ten years to the human life span; radiation protection alone should add two to five years. Success with protein missynthesis resorting should add five to ten years. The three protection mechanisms together will act synergistically, potentially producing a life-span increase of thirty to forty years of youthful life.

—Richard A. Passwater
Supernutrition for Healthy Hearts

SPECIFIC NUTRIENT ANTIOXIDANTS

In addition to the body's natural antioxidant production, oral antioxidants are able to be utilized efficaciously to protect against oxidative processes. These include vitamins E, C, and A; beta-carotene; selenium–glutathione; cysteine-methionine; ubiquinone; riboflavin; zinc, copper, and manganese; and dimethylglycine. The following descriptions, contributed by Karuna Corp. in northern California, describes some of the qualities of these oral antioxidants.

VITAMIN E (TOCOPHEROL)

Tocopherols protect highly unsaturated fatty acids in lipid membranes from the effect of molecular oxygen. Vitamin E is in the chain-breaking group of antioxidants. The tocopherols are phenols which are able to trap peroxyl radicals by transferring the phenolic hydrogen, forming a relatively unreactive phenoxyl radical that is either destroyed by reaction with a second peroxyl radical or is reduced to the starting phenol by reaction with vitamin C. Because vitamin E acts to improve red-cell membrane integrity, it has been found effective for patients with beta-thalassemia and sickle-cell anemia. It has been found useful in two conditions in premature infants—retrolental fibroplasia after oxygen respiratory therapy and respiratory distress syndrome. Studies indicate that alpha tocopherols have three times the antioxidant effect of gamma tocopherols in preventing iron-induced free-radical formation. The activity of glutathione peroxidase has been found to be very low, not only in selenium-deficient animals, but in those with vitamin E deficiency as well. An Israeli study reported on the effectiveness of vitamin E in the treatment of osteoarthritis. Along with selenium, it has been found to have a protective effect against ischemic heart-tissue damage resulting from various cardiovascular problems. Vitamin E has been found to inhibit arachidonic acid-induced platelet aggregation. These are but a few of the antioxidant-related functions reported in the literature for vitamin E.

SELENIUM–GLUTATHIONE

Selenium is an essential component of glutathione peroxidase, the enzyme that destroys hydroperoxides by using the reducing equivalents of reduced glutathione. Thus, it is difficult to separate the antioxidant effects of the two. A selenium deficiency has been linked to an increased toxicity from polycyclic hydrocarbons, many of which are carcinogenic and mutagenic. Another investigation found reduced glutathione to be an effective protector against bladder damage incurred by treatment with alkylating anti-tumor drugs, as well as in treatment of aflatoxin-B-induced liver tumors. Further studies have indicated the inability of selenium-deficient hearts to metabolize hydroperoxides via glutathione-dependent pathways. Selenium supplementation in high doses in animals appears to be a therapeutic agent for the treatment of Erlich ascites tumors. In general, selenium is one of the most potent broad-spectrum anticarcinogenic agents yet discovered, and when added to food and water of animals at a concentration of 1–4 parts per million provides protection against many carcinogenic agents.

BETA CAROTENE–VITAMIN A

Beta carotene, although an antioxidant, does not employ conventional mechanisms. It scavenges free radicals at low oxygen partial pressures only. These low oxygen pressures are found in most tissues under normal physiological conditions. It thus complements vitamin E, which has its effect at higher oxygen concentrations. Reports indicate that beta carotene inhibits xanthine oxidase-initiated lipid peroxidation. It has been shown to quench singlet oxygen, which is produced during photo-oxidation reactions, which may directly peroxidize unsaturated fats. Beta carotene seems to have a substantial protective effect against lung cancer in smokers.

Vitamin A is a fat-soluble antioxidant. Studies indicate its protective effect against enhanced lipid peroxidation by ethanol and carbon tetrachloride.

VITAMIN C

Vitamin C is a water-soluble antioxidant, which exists in the interstitial fluid where it acts on the external cell membrane or in the cytoplasm, where it protects external mitochondrial, endoplasmic reticulum and microsomal membranes. It readily accepts electrons and serves as a free-radical scavenger. It appears to protect against the peroxidative effects of ethanol and carbon tetrachloride. As previously mentioned, it has the power to return the tocopherols in the form of phenoxyl radical to their reduced phenolic form. Case studies cite a protective role for vitamin C with regard to gastric cancer. It is a well-known inhibitor of nitrosamine formation, nitrosamines having been linked to cancer of the esophagus and gastrointestinal tract. Another study demonstrated regression of adenomatous rectal polyps in a group of patients on 3 grams of vitamin C a day. Increased risks of cardiovascular disease, particularly in regard to thrombosis, have been linked to low leukocyte and platelet levels of various antioxidants, including vitamin C as well as selenium and vitamin E. Vitamin C has been found to strongly oppose platelet aggregation. Like selenium and vitamin E, vitamin C has been found to protect adriamycin-treated animals from cardiotoxicity, a dangerous side effect of this anti-tumor drug.

CYSTEINE–METHIONINE

Methionine is an essential amino acid. Cysteine is produced from methionine. Only the L-forms of these amino acids are biologically active. Cysteine is an important component of glutathione and both are water-soluble antioxidants. Animal studies indicate that lung glutathione levels correlate directly with the levels of sulphur-containing amino acids, cysteine and methionine, in their diets. Oxygen tolerance in animals has been found to decrease when protein-deficient states are induced. Experiments reveal a protective effect from oxygen toxicity in this situation by addition of cysteine and methionine in the diet. Acetaminophen toxicity in humans, both acute and chronic, has been effectively treated by the antioxidant effects of N-acetylcysteine, L-methionine as well as vitamin E and glutathione. Cysteine has been found to be effective in treating the toxic effects of alkylating free radicals produced by ipomeanol metabolites such as are found in moldy potatoes.

UBIQUINONE (CO-ENZYME Q)

Ubiquinone is a lipid-soluble, electron carrying co-enzyme. It is an important component of the mitochondrial respiratory chain. Mitochondria peroxidize readily in vitro due to their high content of polyunsaturated fats. Ubiquinone has been found to protect mitochondria from this peroxidation. Its effect seems to be due not only to a reaction with free radicals but also to a membrane-stabilizing effect on the lipid bi-layer. Ubiquinone has been found useful in the prevention of antioxidant deficiency symptomatology and, like others, it reduces the cardiotoxicity of adriamycin as well as the hepatotoxicity of ethanol and carbon tetrachloride. It has been found to provide therapeutic benefit in congestive heart failure, essential hypertension, and periodontal disease as well as having immunostimulating qualities.

EVIDENCE THAT MORE IS BETTER

A new study on congestive heart disease patients showed that doses of 200-300 mg a day of coenzyme Q10 produced significantly better results than previously used doses of 30-150 mg a day.

Dr. Karl Folkers, who has devoted his life to studying CoQ10, has recently stated that the epidemic of congestive heart failure is probably the result of a deficiency of CoQ10. Based on CoQ10's mechanism of action, heart muscle cells would derive enormous benefit by having access to the optimal level of energy-producing coenzyme Q10.

In the July 1994 issue of the popular Health and Healing newsletter, Dr. Julian Whitaker reported that high doses of CoQ10 appeared to be very effective in treating advanced cancer patients. Anecdotal reports showed impressive results in treating metastatic lung and stomach cancers. One study published in Biochemical and Biophysical Research Communications showed that a combination of vitamins, minerals, and high doses of CoQ10 produced statistically significant results in treating breast cancer patients. Dose ranges were 90 mg to 390 mg a day of CoQ10 with the higher doses producing better results.

CoQ10's mechanism of action in treating cancer is partially due to its ability to boost immune function, but the regression of these cancers indicate that there may be additional antineoplastic mechanisms associated with high doses of CoQ10.

—Life Extension Foundation

RIBOFLAVIN 5–PHOSPHATE

Riboflavin (Vitamin B_2) is an essential component of the antioxidant system. The flavin nucleotides, FMN and FAD, function as prosthetic groups on numerous enzymes involved in oxidation-reduction reactions as well as electron transport. It is important for the proper function of glucose-6-phosphate dehydrogenase, a glutathione-sparing enzyme involved in the oxidation and reduction of glutathione.

ZINC, COPPER, AND MANGANESE

Zinc and copper are important components of the cytosol form of superoxide dismutase while manganese is found in mitochondrial superoxide dismutase. Deficiencies of these minerals have been found to lower the activity of their respective superoxide dismutases. A number of different copper chelates have been found to have antioxidant and anti-inflammatory activity. Zinc deficiency has been found to reduce glutathione levels and interfere with selenium metabolism. A manganese deficiency may result in a five-fold increase in lipid peroxidation and subsequent mitochondrial membrane damage.

SOME PLANT AND ANIMAL ANTIOXIDANT SOURCES

almond	vitamin E
apricot	beta carotene
beef	zinc
broccoli	beta carotene, vitamin C, selenium
cantaloupe	beta carotene, vitamin C
carrot	beta carotene
cauliflower	vitamin C
celery	selenium
cheese, milk products	zinc
citrus fruits	vitamin C
cucumber	selenium
filbert	vitamin E, zinc
fish	selenium, zinc
garlic	selenium
grains	vitamin E, selenium
green pepper	vitamin C
honeydew	vitamin C
kale	beta carotene, vitamin E
legumes	zinc
liver	zinc
lobster	selenium
mushroom	selenium
oyster	zinc
peach	beta carotene
peanut	vitamin E, zinc
pecan	vitamin E, zinc
poultry	zinc
pumpkin	beta carotene
red pepper	vitamin C
shrimp	vitamin E, selenium
spinach	beta carotene, vitamin E
strawberry	vitamin C
sweet potato	vitamin E
tomato	vitamin C
vegetable oils	vitamin E
watermelon	vitamin C
wheat germ	vitamin E
winter squash	beta carotene

DIMETHYLGLYCINE

As a potent methyl donor, dimethylglycine improves oxygen utilization by the cell. It improves circulation as well as oxygen uptake by the heart. It also supports detoxification by the liver, perhaps by donating methyl groups to potentially toxic substances, rendering them harmless. It is also used to form methionine, the importance of which has been discussed.

There is evidence that a deficiency of even one of the important components of the antioxidant system may result in increased oxidative damage. Thus, it appears that they all work synergistically to help prevent the development of degenerative disease that may result from long-term oxidative damage.

REJUVENATION

To go beyond the maximum limit that is imposed by metabolic aging, we must look deeper into the genetics of the cell and into a process known as mitosis—cell division. When a cell divides properly it completely regenerates itself. Therein lies the key to the reversal and ultimate control of aging. Controlling excess free-radical damage supports cellular health and maintenance, and thus provides an environment conducive to the continuation of healthy mitosis.

CHAPTER SIX

OTHER THEORIES OF AGING

Various theories of reversing aging can be viewed as related to either the life-extension or regeneration approaches. The free-radical theory of aging, presented in depth in the previous chapter, shows great promise as a breakthrough in understanding aging on the cellular level. Some of the other widely known theories of aging will be reviewed in this chapter to provide an introduction to the theoretical science as a foundation for practical applications that benefit individual health.

Biological systems of the various organs of the body are better preserved when the maximum life span is significantly extended. This leads to the conclusion that all systems of the body age although in different ways and at different rates. As Vincent Cristofalo so aptly phrased it, aging is "a multifactorial process composed of both genetic and environmental components. Each physiologic system within an organism, each tissue within a system, and each cell type within a tissue appears to have its own trajectory of aging."

Nutrient-rich caloric restriction has been shown to slow aging in all biological systems. It does not reverse aging, although in humans, dramatic physiological changes as a result of caloric restriction, such as reduction in hypertension, inhibit or prevent many common illnesses that cause premature aging and even death. The cure of aging, at its most fundamental level, will most likely have to come on the cellular level, by methods that reactivate cell division.

THEORIES OF AGING

SOMATIC-MUTATION THEORY

One somatic-mutation theory of aging postulates that random genetic damage occurs from environmental radiation. The source of radiation could be the sun, pollution, power lines, appliances, and office equipment. Such damage causes errors in the synthesis of proteins and induces cancers. The accumulation of such damage over time is what we observe as aging.

Radiation does cause such degenerative processes. In an environment free of radiation, however, animals continue to age and die essentially along the same survival curve as animals in normal environments. It seems that the damage from environmental radiation is not the fundamental cause of aging.

According to Finch and Hayflick in their book *The Handbook of the Biology of Aging*, other models concerning somatic mutation as a cause of aging include somatic mutation as the result of intrinsic mutagenesis at the time of division, and a time-dependent mutagenesis in resting cells. Experiments need to be performed to test the validity of these hypotheses.

DNA-REPAIR THEORY OF AGING

The DNA-repair theory postulated by scientists R. W. Hart and R. B. Setlow originates from observations that the DNA of various species with different life spans have different levels of repair. The species with the longer life spans have a greater level of repair. Current research, however, does not find much difference in the level of DNA repair among young and old of the same species. Results of experiments have not been announced in which DNA repair has been artificially enhanced to see if the maximum life span is increased.

REPAIR AND LIFE SPAN

Hart and Setlow grew primary fibroblast cultures out of the dermis of several species. The cultures were irradiated. . .Most active in repair were human, elephant, and cow fibroblasts. They were nearly 5 times as active as the fibroblasts of rats, mice, or shrews. . . .

Repair capability and life span are not proportional. Man, for example, lives 25 times as long as a rat, not 5 times. Results do suggest that long-lived species may have more active repair systems and that their excision systems might also be more sophisticated in detecting a broader spectrum of injury.

—Caleb E. Finch and Leonard Hayflick
The Handbook of the Biology of Aging

ERROR-CATASTROPHE THEORY OF AGING

In the normal operation of the cell, errors occur in DNA and RNA, the templates for protein synthesis. Those templates, once altered, then proceed to transcribe error-containing molecules. One hypothesis is that the accumulation of such erroneous molecules inevitably leads to cell aging and death. Although there is missynthesis of proteins in normal metabolism, however, it does not seem to be related to age. Most of the protein damage seems to occur by oxidative processes such as free-radical reactions or in a process called glycation, wherein surplus glucose is incorporated into protein construction.

CROSS-LINKAGE THEORY OF AGING

DNA and protein structures become excessively cross-linked in the normal metabolic process. This happens both within the cell itself and also in the extracellular matrix, with connective tissue being the prime target. Over time, the accumulation of cross-linked molecules causes the malfunction of biological processes and aging. This theory (that aging is caused by cross-linkage of the DNA and protein molecules) dovetails with the error-catastrophe theory and the free-radical theory. Cross-linkage can be caused by normal oxidative and glycation processes.

NEUROENDOCRINE THEORIES OF AGING

A cluster of theories of aging exist, proposing that deterioration in certain groups of neurons and the hormones with which they are associated is a major cause of aging. The central hypothesis is the deterioration of a three-way system involving the hypothalamus, the pituitary, and the adrenal glands. The neuroendocrine system regulates early development, growth, puberty, the reproductive system, menopause, and metabolism, and it is involved in most physiological functions. Obviously, deterioration of this biochemical central-processing unit has general repercussions. Attempts to compensate for deficits in endocrine functions with Melatonin and pineal polypeptal extract have improved average life span and increased maximum life span. It can also increase quality of life. The supplementation of growth hormone, estrogen, testosterone, and the adrenal hormone dehydroepiandrosterone (DHEA), all of which decline with age, does not seem to significantly improve the normal survival curve.

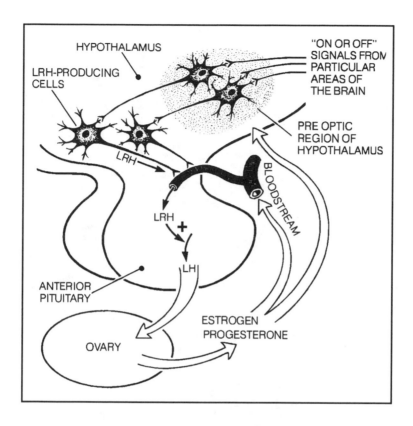

Figure 6.1 Brain Regulation of Estrogen & Progesterone in the Bloodstream & Tissues

In this diagram, estrogen and progesterone are used as examples to show a process generally true for hormones. The cells in the preoptic region of the hypothalamus collect information from other regions of the brain and act as "timers" or cycle regulators. When activated, these nerve cells stimulate cells that produce LRH (luteinizing hormone-releasing hormone), which is secreted into the blood that enters the pituitary gland. In the pituitary, the LRH activates the production of LH (luteinizing hormone), which goes by the bloodstream to the ovary, where it turns on production of estrogen and progesterone. Estrogen and progesterone then act at specific target organs (uterine cells) and on the brain. In the brain, these steroids affect the system which started their synthesis and regions that influence sexual behavior. This chain of events shows one route by which the mental state is translated into hormone chemistry.

From *Secrets of Life Extension* by John Mann. Used by permission.

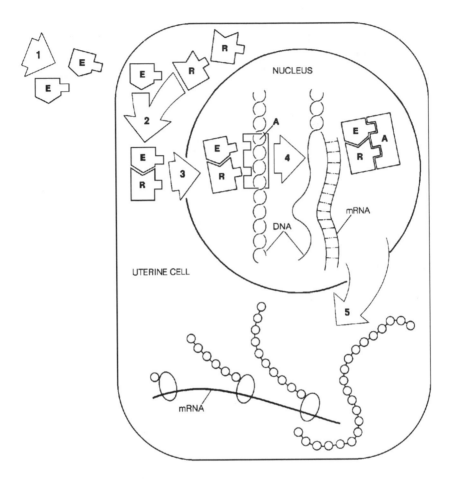

Figure 6.2 How a Steroid Hormone Works in the Cell

The mechanism shown here has been found to be true for many hormones; here estrogen is used as an example. The hormone (E) circulates in the bloodstream, but concentrates in certain target cells, here the uterine cell. A special protein called a receptor (R) binds the estrogen molecule in a lock-and-key fashion. This complex moves into the nucleus, and by matching with a specific acceptor protein (A) associated with the "estrogen genes" causes that part of the DNA to be copied to mRNA. The mRNA then moves to the cytoplasm for translation to protein, and the cellular changes characteristic of estrogen response start. The role of the hormone, then, is to act directly to switch on a special DNA-to-mRNA transcription.

From *Secrets of Life Extension* by John Mann. Used by permission.

HORMONE-REPLACEMENT THERAPY

Hormone-replacement therapy can be of undisputed value if certain steroids are in short supply because of age or illness. The anabolic nature of the steroids can assist tissue building in people who are rundown from these or other causes....

Hormonal therapy is most effective when all other factors contributing to health and youth preservation are in order; e.g., diet, mental and neuronal health, adequate exercise, proper rest, and sufficient exposure to sunlight....

Hormonal replacement therapy should be given only with natural steroids or exact synthetic replicas of these. Self-administration should never be attempted. Such therapy should not even be conducted by an ordinarily good physician, but rather by a competent endocrinologist with the best modern monitoring facilities available.

—John Mann
Secrets of Life Extension

Hormonal supplementation is a high profile type of therapy that receives a lot of attention. The following article recently appeared in a national newspaper. The names have been redacted because the point is not to criticize the people but rather the way the information is presented.

TESTOSTERONE MAY WARD OFF MEN'S AGING

Extra doses of testosterone show "promise" of reversing some bad effects of aging in men over 50, a new study says.

Injections of the male hormone improved strength, steadied balance, boosted red blood cell counts (to stave off anemia) and lowered cholesterol, says Dr. X of the ABC University Medical School. She presented findings at the Y Society meeting in Anytown, USA over the weekend.

Some studies have suggested that testosterone might fuel growth of prostate cancer. Researchers do not yet know how testosterone injections will affect that risk.

Dr. X selected 21 men, ranging in age from their 50s to their 80s, with below-average levels of the hormone. Semi-weekly testosterone shots were given to 10, and 11 got placebos. After six months:

- Men on the hormone had significantly larger muscles and better strength, and also were significantly stronger than those given placebos.
- Men taking the hormone also had higher red blood cell counts and lower cholesterol.

Another payoff: better sex. "For those getting the testosterone, they and their wives really knew it," Dr. X says.

—**Summary of Associated Press Wire Story**

There is a common fallacy in the above report. Perhaps the reporter does not understand the nuances of aging research. It is possible that the researcher does not understand the misconception. Note that the article mentions that men "with below-average levels of the hormone" were selected. Below-average levels of *anything* important will deplete the body and cause it to deteriorate at an accelerated rate. Supplementing back the deficient element may revitalize the subject. But what does this have to do with aging in normal people. All too often, this type of article leads people to think that if you just had some testosterone, or whatever agent is being discussed, that you would gain "larger muscles" and "better strength" such that your wife "really knew it." The truth of the matter is that "normal" aging males are deficient in testosterone. Yet if a hormone is supplemented when it is not needed, the glands may cut back on natural production of that hormone and health and vitality suffer as a result.

IMMUNOLOGIC THEORY OF AGING

The functional vitality of the immune system does decline with age. The immune system's response to infection is diminished with age. The incidence of cancer, which is under immunologic control, increases with age. With aging there is also an increasing incidence of autoimmune reactions. All of these factors support the idea that damage to tissue from infection, toxicity, and attacks by the immune system on the self are major causes of aging. However, the survival curves of animals raised in completely sterile environments is essentially the same as animals who are maintained in unhygienic environments. This would indicate that while there is decline in immune status, it is not central to aging. Also, artificially dampening the immune system does not seem to increase life span. Thus, autoimmune reactions do not seem to be the major factor in normal aging.

Functional deterioration in specialized systems of the body does not seem to impact much on the overall life span. Therefore the aging of any one system is probably not *the* cause of aging.

THEORIES OF AGING

The theories of aging presented in this chapter encapsulate a few of the more widely known theories of aging under close scrutiny within the scientific communities of the world. Various theories of aging will be presented, examined, and either proven or disproven over the course of time since thousands of researchers have attempted and will continue to attempt to discover the secrets of the fountain of youth. So far, a nutrient-dense regimen of caloric restriction shows the most promise toward retarding the process of aging, but only time will tell what other secrets will be revealed.

CHAPTER SEVEN

AGING AND THE BIOLOGICAL SYSTEMS

This chapter focuses on the aging of particular biological systems. In each of us some organ groups age or deteriorate more rapidly than others. In order to age more healthfully, we should learn the practical approaches to preserve these systems.

THE CARDIOVASCULAR SYSTEM

The cardiovascular system includes the heart and the vessels by which blood is pumped and circulated through the body, the veins and arteries. Nutrients and hormones are delivered to all tissues via the cardiovascular system. Immune cells and oxygen-carrying cells navigate through the body via the blood. Waste products are carried away by the blood. While all biological systems are critical, the vascular system deserves the most immediate attention. Two diseases of this system, heart attack and stroke, comprise about 60 percent of all deaths, a good portion of which may be premature and preventable. Studies show that the leading cause for death for humans age 45 and older is arteriosclerosisor hardening of the blood vessels.

The aging of the cardiovascular system should be viewed as a complex, highly selective process that warrants individualized diagnosis and management. A primary focus should be on the prevention of heart disease. Causes of heart disease include inadequate coronary blood supply, anatomical disorders, and arrhythmias. Diseases of the cardio-vascular system include hypertension, arteriosclerosis, heart attack, and stroke.

The following changes appear to characterize normal physiologic aging. The cardiac mass, or weight of the heart related to body weight, increases while the cardiac efficiency decreases. Hypertrophy, or en-largement, of the heart is accompanied by a change in the enzymatic property of myosin, which is the main protein in muscle. Simulta-neously, the walls of the greater arteries become thicker, more rigid, and less pliant. At the same time, the collagen fraction and the amount of collagen-bound calcium increases. The elastic component decreases, at least relatively, and the elastin-collagen ratio clearly diminishes with age.

These alterations are similar to those observed in the disease of arterial hypertension. The arterial hypertension most probably is the primary pathology rather than the aging. These changes result in decrease in blood-vessel permeability, the ability to allow oxygen and nutrients through the walls of the blood vessels. These changes also facilitate the accumulation of fat and proteinaceous compounds from blood plasma and constitute a link between aging and process of arteriosclerosis. Prevention of hypertension and arteriosclerosis could retard the physical symptoms of cardiovascular aging.

HYPERTENSION

Hypertension, or high blood pressure, is caused by the malfunc-tioning of one or more organs that maintain normal blood pressure. These malfunctions may include the heart pumping excess blood, the kidneys excreting too much blood, a high level of hormones capable of increasing blood pressure, and constriction of the blood vessels. Effects of hypertension include enlargement of the heart itself due to working harder by pumping more blood, and consequent weakening of the heart muscle due to such exertion; arteriosclerosis; and organ damage or failure. High blood pressure is considered dangerous at any age. Treating high blood pressure is essential.

ARTERIOSCLEROSIS

Atherosclerosis is the disease of the intima of the arteries that leads to fatty lesions. Arteriosclerosis is the degenerative disease commonly known as "hardening of the arteries," when the arteries become thickened and weakened with consequent reduction of permeability. Recent research shows that the end result of arteriosclerosis is actually bone growth within the blood vessels.

WHAT CAUSES ARTERIES TO HARDEN:

UCLA Researchers Find Tiny Slivers of Bone

Hardening of the arteries, long known as a sign of heart attack danger, is exactly what it sounds like—microscopic slivers of actual bone grow in the blood vessel linings, UCLA researchers report.

The bony deposits, or calcifications, are an end result of inflammation in the artery walls due to fat-rich substances often called "bad cholesterol," known medically as low-density lipoproteins.

The microscopic bits of bone pose a definite danger. Coupled with inflammation where new arterial deposits are forming, the stiff spurs can rip open the delicate inner linings of arteries, stimulating sudden formation of blood clots.

Once under the layer of cells lining arteries, the fat-like globules of low-density lipoproteins become chemically altered by a process called oxidation. Many take a form that mimics the outer membrane of common bacteria, including the organism that causes tuberculosis and, in the lungs, causes formation of bone-like calcium deposits.

Cells in the artery, reacting against the low-density lipoprotein molecules, signal for help from the body's disease-fighting
monocytes, types of white blood cells. The result is a swelling on
the artery wall. In addition, chemical released in the inflammatory reaction turn on genes for bone formation. When fighting
bacteria, such hard deposits may help wall an infection off from
the rest of the body, but bone does not belong in arteries.

The stiff, bone-reinforced segments of artery walls then may
crack, bringing blood from inside the artery into contact with
the inflammation [resulting in a blood clot].

—Charles Petit

San Francisco Chronicle

HEART ATTACK

Heart attack occurs when a segment or branch of the coronary
artery, the blood vessel that feeds the heart, is blocked. Blockage is
usually caused by a narrowing of the blood vessel by an atheroma, a
localized accumulation of fatty or calcified material on the interior
surface of the vessel. The atheroma increases in size over time. It can
cause the blockage or, more frequently, a blood clot catches in the
narrowed artery.

Usually the condition of poor circulation to the heart is signaled
well in advance of an actual attack. An early symptom includes short-
ness of breath upon moderate exertion. In a more advanced stage of the
disease process, one symptom may be prolonged heavy pressure or
squeezing pain in the center of the chest behind the breastbone. This
chest pain may radiate to the shoulder, neck, arm, fourth and fifth
fingers of the left hand, or to the jaw. The symptoms may be intermit-
tent.

If any symptoms are present, a physician may order such tests as an
electrocardiogram and blood chemistry. If the findings are negative,
sometimes nitroglycerin is prescribed. Nitroglycerin rapidly dilates the
coronary arteries and is most often used in the treatment of chest pain
associated with cardiac insufficiency. If there is a subsequent episode of

chest pain, and nitroglycerin is taken and the pain does not diminish, then the pain is probably caused by something other than the lack of circulation to the heart. If the nitroglycerin does cause the chest pain to recede, then further diagnostic cardiology is probably warranted. The nitroglycerin may cause a transient and insignificant headache as a side effect, because the vessels to the brain are also expanded, causing a change in blood pressure.

STROKE

When a blockage or rupture of a blood vessel interrupts the supply of blood to the brain, the result is the death of nerve cells. This condition is known as a cerebral vascular accident, or stroke. Depending upon the extent, severity, and location of the damage to the brain, symptoms of stroke vary, and may include dizziness, slurred speech, loss of muscular control, diminution or loss of sensation or consciousness, and paralysis. A stroke is the main cause of disability in adults.

WARNING SIGNS OF STROKE

1. Sudden blurred or decreased vision in one or both eyes.
2. Numbness, weakness, or paralysis of the face, or in either an arm or a leg, on one side or both sides of the body.
3. Difficulty in speaking or understanding.
4. Dizziness, loss of balance, or an unexplained fall.
5. Difficulty in swallowing.
6. Headache that is severe and comes on abruptly, or unexplained changes in a pattern of headaches.

These symptoms are usually temporary, and last from a few seconds up to twenty-four hours. You may think you have recovered. . .[but] these temporary interruptions, known as TIAs (transient ischemic attacks), are serious warning signs of stroke. Contact your doctor immediately.

—Bradley Gascoigne, M.D.
Smart Ways to Stay Young and Healthy

Factors Causing Heart Disease and Stroke

The main factors that cause heart disease and stroke can be viewed as a set of conditions: high blood pressure over a period of many years, excess fat in the body, elevated serum cholesterol and other lipoproteins, a diet high in salt, protein, and fat, lack of proper physical exercise, and chronically elevated adrenal hormones associated with emotional anxiety. Individuals vary considerably.

LIFESTYLE CHANGES THAT HELP REDUCE HYPERTENSION

- Reduce dietary salt, fat, and protein
- Keep body weight close to optimal
- Maintain physical exercise including jogging, swimming, or power walking
- Avoid toxic substances including cigarettes, alcohol, caffeine, solvents, pesticides, and pollution
- Manage emotional stress
- Have regular medical evaluations
- If necessary, use medications to control blood pressure and lower serum cholesterol
- Take a baby aspirin daily as an anticoagulant and anti-inflammatory agent

Aging does not appear to be the primary consideration in the decline of the cardiovascular system. Life style and behavior-modification changes can be implemented to help to regain improved cardiovascular function.

ENDOCRINE SYSTEM

The endocrine system encompasses ductless glands that secrete chemical substances, hormones, directly into the blood system. These hormones influence metabolism and other body functions. The hormone-secreting glands are the adrenal glands, the gonads, the islets of Langerhans in the pancreas, the parathyroid glands, the pineal body, the pituitary-adrenal system, the pituitary gland, and the thyroid gland.

Every cell in the body makes most of its own constituent parts within itself. Certain essential components, however, are manufactured by the endocrine glands. These components, hormones, are distributed via the blood. Like nutrients, they are used by individual cells as needed. The body also uses the endocrine glands to communicate biochemically with its different systems. The endocrines are linked to the nervous system and thereby with the external world.

For example, if you see a car about to hit you those visual signals are transferred to your adrenal system, which floods your body with an array of substances that excite virtually everything to move rapidly. While in this instance there is a car actually speeding at you, a similar biological effect can be caused by vivid imagery within one's mind. This phenomenon has opened an intriguing area of investigation called "psychoneuroendocrinimmunology." It may be possible that with guided imagery, we can consciously "talk" to our endocrine system and influence metabolic processes of the body relative to its vitality and various disease processes. At this time, most of this work is speculative.

HORMONAL EXHAUSTION

Frequently, a gland which has been overstimulated for a long period of time will simply become exhausted and cease to turn out its hormonal quota. Often, however, the diminution or cessation of glandular function is caused not by any degeneration of the gland itself, but by a signal from the brain or nervous system. State of mind is profoundly related to glandular health. A happy, tranquil mind is likely to support healthy endocrines. Optimal hormonal secretions, in turn, engender a sound neural and mental state. Stress, on the other hand, may throw endocrine balances awry. The hypothalamus influences the pituitary to influence other glands. The hypothalamus itself can be influenced by such factors as general health, dietary and exercise habits, brain and nerve conditions, atmospheric ionization, and serotonin levels.

There is now considerable evidence that menopause is caused not by any failure in the ability of the ovaries to produce estrogen, but by a signal from the hypothalamic/pituitary axis that directs the ovaries to stop hormone manufacture and ovulation. Joseph Meites at Michigan State University has caused postmenopausal rats to resume estrogen production and ovulation by electrically stimulating particular centers of the brain, and by increasing brain levels of dopamine and norepinephrine.

—A. Rosenfeld

Prolongevity

Aging is associated with a myriad of endocrine and hormonal changes. The mechanisms underlying these changes vary according to the particular gland. The causes of these changes include programmed cell death, autoimmune destruction of the gland, or neoplastic transformation of glandular tissue. Some of the aging deterioration in hormonal secretions are in the circadian and seasonal rhythm. The responsiveness of the hormonal pulses, the transport of the hormones into the cells, and the rates at which they clear also deteriorate. Hormone balance and reactivity is a sensitive interplay between the secreting gland and the receptivity of and utilization of the hormones by the cells.

The general vitality of the endocrine system is maintained, in substantial measure, by physical exercise and caloric restriction. Generally, attempts to reverse or slow aging by supplementing hormones have not yet been proven effective beyond what can be accomplished with nutrition and exercise. However, hormone replacement together with mineral supplementation in women with certain genetic makeup may be effective in preventing premature osteoporosis—more research is necessary. Growth-hormone replacement has been reported to increase muscle mass, skin thickness, and to restore other biomarkers of aging to more youthful levels. Some of these effects can be accomplished with physical exercise. Drawbacks to supplementing growth hormone include it is extremely expensive, there may be side effects, and it is impractical to administer.

DIGESTIVE SYSTEM

The digestive system includes the mouth, salivary glands, tongue, throat, esophagus, stomach, small and large intestines, appendix, rectum and anus, liver, gallbladder, and pancreas. Through the digestive system, food is taken into the body and dismantled into its basic constituent parts. The nutrients in these parts are then delivered to cells via the circulatory system.

CHANGES IN AGING OF THE GASTROINTESTINAL SYSTEM

- A decrease in gastric secretions
- A slowing of the movement of matter through the intestinal tract
- Structural changes in the intestines and pancreas, colorectal motility (bowel movements), the mass of the liver, and the flow of blood to the organs.

The actual functional significance of these changes is variable. During aging, gastrointestinal functions remain relatively intact because of the large reserve capacity of the intestine, pancreas, and liver.

Some clinically important changes in gastrointestinal function with aging include decreased taste sensation, reduced amount of hydrochloric acid in the stomach, and increased liver mass. Also, there appears to be an increase in the absorption of dietary fats, lipids, and whole proteins. The malabsorption of nutrients is associated with atrophic gastritis, a disease process, rather than aging.

Reducing the amount of food to be processed lowers stress on the digestive system. Routine physical exercise enhances motility and blood flow. Life-extension doctors often recommend food rotation and testing for allergic sensitivity to certain foods. Routine supplementation of digestive enzymes is unnecessary for most people.

EAT FIVE FRUITS OR VEGETABLES A DAY

Nutritional advice used to be fairly straightforward: eat three square meals a day and get the recommended daily amounts (RDAs) of vitamins and minerals. There were the four basic food groups (dairy, meats, fruits and vegetables, and breads and cereals), and you were supposed to reasonably divide your intake among them. But with the high rates in this country of strokes, elevated blood pressures, and heart attacks, concern has arisen about our diets, which are often high in animal fat, overly salted, preservative-laden, artificially colored, and increasingly processed. . . . To show how far nutritional thinking has changed [in the last decade], in the spring of 1991 the Physician's Committee for Responsible Medicine proposed replacing the four food groups with a new four: vegetables, grains, legumes, and fruits.

—Bradley Gascoigne, M.D.
Smart Ways to Stay Young and Healthy

IMMUNE SYSTEM

The immune system involves both cellular and molecular components. The function of the immune system is to distinguish "self" from "nonself" and defend the body against foreign organisms or substances. During the very early stages of development, including up to perhaps several months after birth, the immune system has memorized all the different tissues in the body. Then, rather suddenly, it stops that memorization or encoding process. From that time forward anything in the body that the immune system does not recognize is attacked. The immune system attacks foreign organisms such as bacteria and viruses as well as foreign materials such as pesticides and constituents from food. It also attacks the body's own cells if they mutate or become cancerous.

The bone marrow, thymus gland, spleen, and lymphatic system comprise the major organs of the immune system. The various cells produced by these organs and glands are usually white in color and thus are called leukocytes (*leukos*=clear, white; *cyt*=cell). Types of leukocytes include lymphocytes, macrophages, B cells, and T cells. T cells originate in the thymus. B cells mature in the bone marrow. The T cells' purpose is to alert the B cells to produce antibodies to attack specific invading antigens. These antibodies attach to invading antigens similarly as pieces in jigsaw puzzles fit together. Once joined together, the antigens can be destroyed by the antibodies if the immune system is functioning properly.

WAGING WAR ON THE MOLECULAR LEVEL

All immune system cells are leukocytes, which journey to different parts of the body as they mature. Some white blood cells stay in the circulating blood, some migrate to the lymphatic fluid, and others set up housekeeping in organs or glands. Finally, some of these immune cells travel to the lymphatic areas, where they mature and then later rejoin the general circulation.

This system would be totally chaotic except that the immune cells can communicate with each other, with the brain, and with the cells that are housed in other organs or tissues. These data are delivered by chemical messenger cells, which coordinate the actions and interactions of white blood cells as they wage the immune battle. The leukocytes can be identified by individually coded molecules on their surface. The actions and interactions of all these cells together make up the immune system.

—Gary Null and Martin Feldman, M.D.
Reverse the Aging Process Naturally

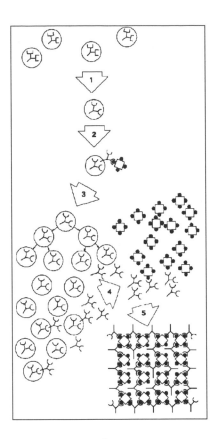

Figure 7.1 Immune and Autoimmune Response

The antibody protein is actually "Y"-shaped, with each of the two arms working as the "locks" for which the antigen carries the "key." The antigen molecule may also have more than one "key" area per molecule; so long chains and networks form when many "locks" are matched with many "keys." (1) An autoimmune response can result if some change in the antibody-producing cell results in an antibody with an altered "lock." (2) If this new "lock" fits a "key" which happens to be part of the normal body, (3) cell division is stimulated as if in response to a foreign antigen. The increased population of the cell then produces large amounts of the altered antibody, and (4) the antibody system is then attacking the "normal" molecules of its own body as if they were the original foreign antigen. (5) As before, the attacked molecules may form a large network.

From *Secrets of Life Extension* by John Mann. Used by permission.

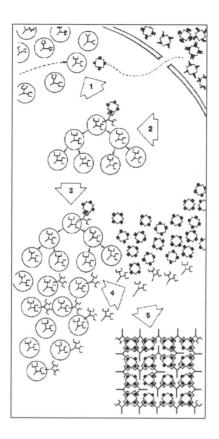

Figure 7.2 Immunologic Memory

(1) An antigen is recognized as a foreign material by a cell which already has a matching "lock" to the antigen "key." (2) This cell is stimulated to divide and produce a clone of that cell. (3) Years later, if one of these selected cells encounters the same antigen, the cell reacts to the antigen, and cell division is stimulated. (4) This produces an increase in the population of that cell, and enough antibodies can be produced to cope with larger amounts of the antigen. These antibodies are proteins which can circulate in the bloodstream and can act at a place far from the cells that produced them. (5) If the antigen has two or more sites at which the antibody can bind, a large network will form, immobilizing the antigen until the body removes the mass.

From *Secrets of Life Extension* by John Mann. Used by permission.

The body is constantly under massive attack by foreign organisms and toxic substances. Any aging in the immune system would have detrimental repercussions for all the other tissues in the body. The study of all aspects of immunity has received a major impetus due to funding for research on Acquired Immune Deficiency Syndrome (AIDS), also known as HIV (Human Immunodeficiency Virus) disease. AIDS is an accelerated model of what might be happening during normal aging.

AIDS is apparently a disease associated with a particular type of retrovirus. This retrovirus either switches off the proper surveillance of some immune functions or causes the immune system to destroy itself by an autoimmune response. A person with HIV disease experiences an accelerated decline in general vitality, increasing inability to fend off infection, and high susceptibility to certain cancers. These are symptoms that occur during aging, but over a longer period of time than in someone with active AIDS whose demise is most probably certain and relatively fast.

The aging of the immune system causes the individual to be more vulnerable to many infections, lowers resistance to toxic substances, and increases susceptibility to cancer and autoimmune diseases. The important functional changes appear particularly in the T-cell functions.

The rapidly emerging field of biotechnology is producing new methods of modulating immune function, with ever-increasing specificity. The future holds promise for restoring immunologic function, whether dysfunction is caused by disease or is part of the aging process. Most of this work, however, is still being conducted at the level of basic experimental science.

Roy Walford, who could be said to be the father of the immune theory of aging, has turned to caloric restriction as a way to improve immune system functioning during aging. With caloric restriction, the incidence of cancer is dramatically reduced, response to infection is improved, and most parameters of immunologic function are better maintained.

The medicinal property of many botanicals is currently under scientific investigation to aid in the stimulation of a healthy immune system. The following phytogenic plants are currently being researched.

HERBS TO ENHANCE THE IMMUNE SYSTEM

Echinacea. This plant increases the number of B cells and plasma cells, enhancing the production of antibodies to invaders such as bacteria, viruses, and toxins. Echinacea also activates phagocytes and potentiates the functioning of macrophages, the immune cells that engulf bacteria, fungi, parasites, and tumors. Finally, it stimulates the "complement" system, which works with the immune system to neutralize toxins and carry out other immune functions.

Astragalus. By increasing antibodies this herb helps to fight specific bacteria, viruses, and toxins. Astragalus also stimulates interferon, the chemical that helps to inhibit viruses, and increases both the volume and the activity of phagocytes and macrophages. Finally, it enhances the transformation of T4 cells. As a result the T-helper cells (a T4 subtype) can assist the functioning of B cells, macrophages, natural killer cells, and T-suppressor cells.

Ligustrum. Ligustrum both increases the number of white blood cells and enhances their functioning. Therefore it has an impact on the B cells, T cells, phagocytes and macrophages, and natural killer cells, all of which fight cells infected with foreign antigens.

Shiitake. This mushroom stimulates immune system cells such as macrophages and T4 cells. (It also activates the complement system to help defend the body against foreign invaders.

Glycyrrhiza. Also known as licorice, this plant's primary immune function is to enhance the production of antibodies. Other studies show that glycyrrhiza promotes macrophage activity and the production of interferon. In test-tube studies it has inhibited the growth of viral invaders such as vaccinia, herpes simplex, and vesicular stomatitis virus. Finally, it may have anti-inflammatory and anti-allergy properties as well.

—Gary Null and Martin Feldman, M.D.
Reverse the Aging Process Naturally

MUSCULAR SYSTEM

The muscular system consists of the skeletal muscles, which are the larger muscles directly attached to the large bones. Contraction of these muscles causes the body to run, lift, and move. The muscular system also includes the muscles of the abdomen, face, rib cage, voice box, jaws and mouth, eyes, and many other specialized constructions.

In many humans, up to about the age of 60-70, there appear to be only small changes in the structure and function of muscle tissue. After the age of seventy there is often an acceleration of aging-associated deterioration that involves biochemical changes, loss of muscle mass, and changes in the size and distribution of muscle fibers. Muscles are postmitotic cells. Under normal conditions they are not capable of division and full regeneration. A large part of the deterioration of muscle tissue after age 70 is probably due to atrophy of the neurons that enable the brain to feel the muscle and that stimulate the muscles to contract. It may be that much of the muscle deterioration is caused by disuse and lack of proper neural stimulation.

Preliminary studies injecting human-growth hormone in older humans has shown increases in muscle strength and size. Some similar results can be achieved by physical conditioning.

The general consensus is that participating in a well-rounded program of physical activity that involves resistance training, flexibility, and cardiovascular conditioning will have a significant beneficial effect on maintaining skeletal muscle function. Some investigators are of the opinion that older individuals adapt to resistive and endurance exercise training in a different fashion than young people. They observe that physical conditioning in younger people results in an increase in the number of mitochondria. In older people the number of mitochondria does not increase—only the size of the mitochondria. This may account for the difference in energy output, reduced physical performance, longer life to get in shape, and reduced time to get out of shape in older people.

NERVOUS SYSTEM

The human nervous system governs the functioning of the entire mammalian body. The nervous system consists of what is known as the central nervous system and the peripheral nervous system. The central nervous system consists of the brain and the spinal cord. The peripheral nervous system links the central nervous system with the rest of the body.

MASTER CONTROL CENTER

The brain is the master control center of your whole body. It consumes 25 percent of all metabolic energy, and the six billion nerve cells it contains make up half the body's total nerve cells. It stimulates motor functions, digestion, growth, and tissue repair; it interprets your sensory experiences and decides which physical and emotional responses to make.

Yet despite this incredible power, your brain constitutes only 2 percent of your body's weight. This makes it highly sensitive: nutritional deficiencies can cause brain imbalances that send shock waves through your entire body, resulting in everything from fatigue and forgetfulness to depression and anxiety.

—Robert Adman
The Amino Revolution

THE CENTRAL NERVOUS SYSTEM

The central nervous system consists of the brain and the spinal cord. The brain consists of a hundred *billion* individual nerves cells known as neurons. This system coordinates the peripheral nervous system and integrates the various components of the body into a coherent system. The central nervous system includes those cognitive functions which we so dearly cherish and call our mind.

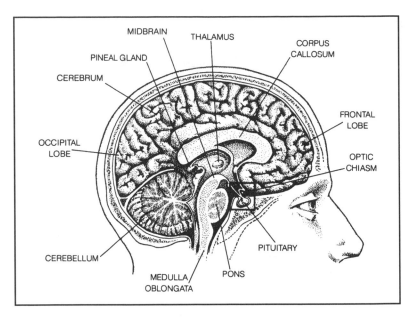

Figure 7.3 The Human Brain: Master Control Center of the Human Body
From *Secrets of Life Extension* by John Mann. Used by permission.

THE PERIPHERAL NERVOUS SYSTEM

The peripheral nervous system connects the central nervous system with the rest of the body. It consists of nerves including the cranial nerves, the spinal nerves, and the sympathetic and parasympathetic nervous systems. The peripheral nervous system is divided into autonomic and somatic functions.

The somatic division of the peripheral nervous system has to do with the body's senses. It includes the cranial and spinal nerves and their ganglia and the all-important peripheral sensory organs that link the body to the outside world.

The autonomic nervous system consists of three subsystems: the enteric, parasympathetic, and sympathetic nervous systems. Generally speaking, the autonomic nervous system regulates the internal processes of the body during both peaceful activity and physical or emotional stress. Autonomic activity is controlled and integrated by the central nervous system, especially those components that receive information relayed from the internal organs.

The enteric nervous system controls the gastrointestinal tract, the pancreas, and the gallbladder. It contains sensory neurons, interneurons, and motor neurons. Thus, the system can sense the tension and the chemical environment in the gut and regulate blood vessel tone, motility, secretions, and fluid transport. The enteric system is itself governed by the central nervous system.

The parasympathetic nervous system generally acts to conserve resources and restore homeostasis, often to balance the sympathetic nervous system.

The sympathetic nervous system mediates the body's response to stressful situations, i.e., the fight or flight reactions. It often acts to balance the parasympathetic system.

The peripheral and central nervous systems constantly interact with each other. At this very moment the written words on this page are creating patterns on the retina of your eye (i.e., your peripheral nervous system), which in turn are inducing pattern recognitions in your cerebral cortex (i.e., your central nervous system).

WEAR AND TEAR ON THE NERVOUS SYSTEM

It is frequently said that we are as old as our nervous system. There is some literal truth to that. The main cell type in the nervous system is the neuron. Neurons are a postmitotic, nondividing type of cell. This means you are working with the same neurons with which you were originally born. With normal metabolism over time, wear and tear results in a decline in the number of neurons as well as in the efficiency of the remaining neurons.

Neurons gradually deteriorate with chronological age because they accumulate damage from the free-radical reactions of normal metabolism. Such damage depletes the functional capacity of the neurons. The damage that occurs to the DNA can result in cell death. When a neuron dies, it is not normally replaced. Because of the progressive accumulation of damage and because of the limitations on the division of neurons, the vitality of the nervous system as a whole declines with age.

A PHENOMENAL NUMBER OF NEURONAL CONNECTIONS

The number of connections made by a single neuron are phenomenal. According to brain researchers, a single neuron can have as many as a hundred thousand synapses connecting it with its neighboring neurons. There may be as many as a hundred billion neurons in the brain–researchers aren't exactly sure how many, though this is a common estimate–the number of connections, reflecting the number of neurons multiplied by the number of synapses, is in the *trillions*.

—Beverly Potter, Ph.D. and Sebastian Orfali
Brain Boosters: Foods & Drugs That Make You Smarter

Neurons and the nervous system remain intact for a much longer time than was previously supposed. When neurological disease is factored out and when arteriosclerosis of the vascular system, which occurs in 90 percent of the population and leads to strokes and diminished brain nutrition, is taken into consideration, the nervous system ages more slowly than other biologic systems.

In early gross anatomical studies, it was noted that brain mass declined with age. For quite a number of years various scientific investigators seemed to confirm that observation. From the measured loss of about 7 to 10 percent of brain weight between the ages of 30-80, a calculation was made that we lose several thousand neurons each day during that period of life. This idea appealed to people and is still commonly believed. Modern studies, however, do not show significant brain weight decline or neuronal loss in healthy adults.

One of the most likely causes of neuronal aging, at its most fundamental level, is oxidative damage to the mitochondrion, the main energy unit of the cell. Oxidative damage can be slowed by caloric restriction and antioxidant application.

Another approach to slowing the effects of intrinsic neuron deterioration is with agents called "proteolytic enzyme inhibitors." Notice that what was just said was "slowing the *effects* of deterioration"–not slowing deterioration.

Proteolytic enzyme inhibitors are agents that inhibit the cell's production of the enzymes used to break down proteins. There are anabolic and catabolic processes in cell metabolism. Cells actively build up their structures and components (anabolism) and actively break down their structures and components (catabolism). Neurons communicate by mean of chemicals called neurotransmitters or biogenic monoamines. Neurons ability to communicate with each other properly depends on their levels of neurotransmitters. As neurons age, their ability to anabolize or produce neurotransmitters declines. Their ability to catabolize or degrade neurotransmitters remains somewhat constant, however. Consequently, the net level of available neurotransmitters declines. This decline in neurotransmitters is associated with all kinds of deficits including depression, lack of energy, cognitive malfunctions, abnormal blood pressure, and structural instability.

A specific monoamine or neurotransmitter that has received a lot of attention is dopamine. Dopamine plays a central role in overall neuromuscular conditions. A particular part of the brain, the substantia nigra, produces dopamine. A significant decline in dopamine production by the substantia nigra, leads to a condition called Parkinson's disease. Parkinson's disease is characterized by muscle tremors that eventually escalate into extreme muscular rigidity and immobilization.

As the brain ages, it produces less dopamine, and eventually everyone could be afflicted, in some measure, with Parkinson's disease. The cause of that is fairly well understood. The enzyme that produces dopamine is called tyrosine hydroxylase. Between ages 15-60 this enzyme decreases by more than 50 percent. Simultaneously, the enzyme that breaks down dopamine, monoamine oxidase, remains at a high level. The net result is a decrease in the amount of dopamine.

There are two approaches to managing this decline. The first approach,, and the one that is most obvious, is to supplement dopamine. That is, in fact, the standard approach to treating advanced Parkinson's. There are side effects from this approach because oral supplementation is a systemic treatment, administering the dopamine to all cells throughout the body.

Another approach is to administer a proteolytic enzyme inhibitor, which blocks the monoamine oxidase from breaking down the dopamine. Thus, dopamine can remain at a higher level. The administration of proteolytic enzyme inhibitors is a new and sophisticated concept. It is one which is now being developed for potential application in a wide spectrum of diseases.

The use of a proteolytic enzyme inhibitor for Parkinson's disease and its further potential use in life extension and control of aging is central to the work of the scientific investigator, Joseph Knoll.

Knoll is a professor of pharmacology at the Semmelweis University of Medicine, Budapest, Hungary. He started his work in this field in the late 1950s. Originally, his interest was "to find a compound possessing both the amphetamine-like psychostimulant effect and the psycho-energetic effect characteristic of the potent MAO (*monoamine oxidase*) inhibitors" without the side effects of those drugs. As his research evolved, he came to focus on a drug called *selegiline*. In addition to its psychostimulant and antidepressant effects, selegiline had a very specific action for the preservation of the substantia nigra, the degradation of which causes Parkinson's disease. Subsequently his form of selegiline (Eldepryl a.k.a. Deprenyl) has been approved by the FDA for use in treating Parkinson's and "senility." Selegiline is currently the treatment of choice for early onset Parkinson's.

Knoll published research in which he reported that selegiline caused, in experimental animals, a very substantial increase of maximum life span and an extension of sexual vigor. Sexual vigor was used as a measure of functional vitality. Other investigators have confirmed these observations in varying degrees.

How might selegiline slow aging and extend the life span? The answer could be something like the following. By specifically inhibiting the activity of type B monoamine oxidase enzyme, which breaks down the neurotransmitter dopamine, the amount of that neurotransmitter is maintained. Consequently, the functions of the dopamine-dependent neural networks are better maintained. This could mean that contingent biological functions are also better maintained and both vitality and life span are extended.

Although the research on selegiline is far from complete, certain individuals over age 50 have initiated trial applications of the drug under controlled conditions. Knoll and others who advocate selegiline for life extension recommend that individuals who are 45 years old take 5 mg. of selegiline three times a week. The Life Extension Foundation cautions in *The Physician's Guide to Life Extension Drugs* that higher doses are less effective and may have undesired side effects. Currently, huge numbers of life-extension enthusiasts follow a similar regimen, under a qualified physician's supervision.

THE CONGESTED BRAIN THEORY

In the 1970s, William Bondareff and Robert Narotzky of the Northwestern University Medical School in Chicago looked inside the brains of rats, at the spaces between the cells. When they measured those spaces, they found that they were only half as wide in older rats as they were in their younger counterparts. It may be that these spaces are akin to Los Angeles freeways, in that they are the "roads" along which travel the vital chemicals that are the brain's messengers. As anyone who lives in Los Angeles knows, when you narrow the freeway, even by one lane, you get horrible traffic jams, and everybody's late to work. It could be that just this sort of thing is going on in the aging brain. And if the messengers—the neurochemicals—get bogged down because of congestion, so does the brain. Since much of the rest of the body needs the brain to tell it what to do when the brain gets jammed, the body has a rough time processing its workload.

—Kathy Keeton
Longevity: The Science of Staying Young

The aging of the nervous system can be slowed by caloric restriction. The acceleration of aging can be countered by preventing or treating hypertension and minimizing exposure to toxic substances, particularly tobacco smoke, alcohol, and the chemicals in an industrial workplace. Physical exercise and recreation enhances and maintains neurological functions. Further, many life-extension enthusiasts experiment with proteolytic enzyme inhibitors such as selegiline. Do not forget that those precious cognitive functions that we call our mind need exercise also. An inactive mind accelerates aging of the physical brain. Mental exercise, puzzles, reading, learning, and recalling knowledge and experiences add more life to our years as well.

However one might slow the aging of the nervous system the ultimate solution will have to come from the controlled growth of new brain cells. This area is on the cutting edge of experimental biology. Because of the large amount of funding for cancer research, in which cell division is a central issue, knowledge about mitosis is accelerating rapidly. No one knows where the research will lead. We can anticipate major breakthroughs in brain-cell proliferation.

RESPIRATORY SYSTEM

The respiratory system includes the lungs, nose, larynx, paranasal sinuses, pleura, and trachea. These organs are involved in the intake of oxygen and the ventilation of "exhaust" gases from the blood.

In the history of modern gerontology, the measurements of the respiratory system were some of the first to be used as biomarkers of aging. Because the performance of the respiratory system involves the integration of many systems, it is believed that the measurement of respiratory system functions better reflects the aging of the whole body than the measurement of other parameters. For example, between ages 30-80, vital capacity declines 50 percent, maximum breathing capacity is reduced 60 percent, and maximum oxygen uptake goes down as much as 70 percent. Many other biological parameters only decline 5 to 10 percent during that period.

The respiratory system is modified in many ways by age. It is particularly vulnerable to damage from environmental factors. The lungs are susceptible to various diseases such as bacterial pneumonia, tuberculosis, and asthma. They are also subject to damage from the accumulation of toxic substances over time, for example as cigarette smoke and airborne pollutants, which may cause bronchitis, emphysema, carcinoma, and interstitial lung disease. However, when disease conditions are factored out and a nondiseased aging population is observed, the respiratory systems show a great reserve function. This allows for a fairly high degree of physical capacity and activity throughout the normal life span.

LIKE CURES LIKE

The heart heals the heart, lung heals lung, spleen heals spleen; *similia similibus curantur* (like cures like).

—Paracelsus
Early sixteenth-century alchemist

SKELETAL SYSTEM

The skeletal system comprises all of the many different types of bone that form the structural framework of the body. Bones store minerals, allow movement, protect tissues and organs, and are involved in the formation of blood cells. The human skeletal system is comprised of over two hundred bones.

Bone can be divided into two kinds of tissue, cortical (outer) and trabecular (innrer). The skeleton is about 80 percent cortical and 20 percent trabecular. Bone density increases during early development and peaks in late adolescence or early adulthood. Thereafter, the bones begin to age. There is a reduction in the material strength and flexibility of bone in both men and women. Between ages 35-70, the cortical bone strength is diminished in bending capacity by about 15 to 20 percent, and the spongy or cancellous bone strength is reduced 50 percent in compression strength. In addition, bone becomes increasingly brittle and fractures more easily.

Osteoporosis is a condition in which the bones become porous and prone to fracture. It is the most common bone disease associated with aging. Because bone density is formed during early development, osteoporosis can be viewed primarily as a disease originating in development but manifesting in later life. Females reach adolescence and adulthood earlier than males. Consequently they have less dense skeletal systems and are more susceptible to bone loss with aging.

Like all other types of cells, bone cells carry on the process of anabolism and catabolism. It is currently hypothesized that bone deterioration in aging is due to an imbalance between these two processes, that catabolism or breakdown exceeds anabolism or remodeling. This could be an area for use of the proteolytic enzyme inhibitors in an attempt to retard catabolic processes and thereby enhance rebuilding.

It is well established that underutilization of bones causes an acceleration of bone loss. An extreme case is astronauts, who evidence marked bone loss in a weightless environment, even when they are in that environment for only a brief time. Weight training, or almost any kind of physical exercise, stimulates an increase in bone density. Supplementation of calcium and vitamin D also helps maintain bone density and strength. For postmenopausal women, sometimes hormone-replacement therapy is indicated, but there may be unwanted side effects, such as increased rates of breast cancer, that need to be taken into consideration.

SKIN

The skin is the largest organ of the body. It has many functions, some of which are not so obvious. The skin is the most important aspect of the immune system because it prevents pathogens and toxins from entering the blood stream. It is the principle regulator of the body's temperature. Skin eliminates waste products, prevents dehydration, and is a reservoir of food and water. The skin is a sense organ. It makes vitamin D with sunshine. In addition, the skin is the mask through which individuals interact with others. Thus, it has a major social function also.

The skin is the most visible organ to show signs of age and deterioration. Any five-year-old child can tell the difference between a 20 year old and a 40 year old simply by the general appearance of the skin. Skin aging is due to changes in the structure and elasticity of the skin over time. It is fundamentally a physiological process, accelerated and exacerbated by the damaging effects of smoking, improper diet, and exposure to ultraviolet radiation.

Basic aging of the skin, at the cellular and molecular level, is caused in large measure by the destruction of the connective tissue components. This may be attributed to the overproduction of proteolytic enzymes. This is another area in which proteolytic enzyme inhibitors might have therapeutic value.

Interestingly, the cells that make the connective tissue, dermal fibroblasts, evidence the Hayflick phenomenon. The Hayflick limit observes that cells seem to have a limit on their regenerative capacity to reproduce themselves through cell division.

A popular method for slowing skin aging that has been receiving a lot of attention for many years is the application of synthetic vitamin A analogs. These ointments go under various names such as retinoic acid and tretinoin. They help to correct atrophy and dysplasia of the epidermis. They stimulate the production of new collagen subepidermally along with the development of new small blood vessels. Mesenchymal dermal cells become more numerous and larger.

There are no miracles here, however. These ointments must be strictly administered in conjunction with a reduction to sun exposure, or used with a sun screen that does not contain benzenes (a potential carcinogen). Although the synthetic vitamin A analogs correct for some of the photo-aging of the skin, they also make the skin more sensitive to ultraviolet radiation.

Because vitamin E, as an antioxidant, may protect body membranes such as skin from light-induced damage, it is a good idea to use vitamin E topically.

A number of studies have examined the association between cigarette smoking and facial wrinkling. The general conclusion is that smoking causes skin wrinkling. Smoking causes smokers to appear unattractive and prematurely old because of decreased capillary and arteriolar blood flow in the skin, thus damaging the connective tissue. Any drug that causes vasoconstriction might do the same thing. Coffee is also suspect!

The routine use of a "moisturizing" cream is often recommended. There is some controversy about the ingredients, however. If you add oil to your skin, it may reduce its own production of natural oil and the skin might actually become dryer. Vegetable-oil based products such as safflower appear to be more beneficial than petroleum-based products. Another possibility is to use a compound that has small amounts of wax, which simply seals the skin rather than oils it.

THE EVOLUTION OF THE HUMAN BODY

The human body has evolved to an intensely complex and sophisticated "machine," with all systems synergistically interactive and apparently in communication with each other on a cellular level. Preserving these biological systems' well being and functionality is the key to a healthy, vibrant future.

CHAPTER EIGHT

TOOLS TO MEASURE AGING AND GENERAL HEALTH

The basis of any science is the ability to quantify and measure the phenomena being researched. Measurement provides data to monitor conditions and directions. If a particular outcome is desired, the ability to measure shows if the goal is being achieved. Evaluating nutritional levels and measuring biological age monitor the efficacy of any life-extension regimen. Some examples of testing batteries available to measure biological aging and general health that have been designed by research centers around the world are presented in this chapter.

The ability to measure biological aging is the basis of both the research and the clinical practice of life extension. In the preceding chapters, some theories about aging and life extension have been presented. Underneath all of that discussion is the issue of measuring biological aging. After decades of research this issue is still far from being resolved.

The aging process can be called a disease—the *one* disease that *everyone* over the age of thirty "catches." There must be some way to diagnose aging, as well as objective means to determine whether the anti-aging treatments utilized are doing any good. Do we feel and perform better? Are the treatments keeping us young longer? Will they extend our life spans?

One way to answer these questions would be to study humans the same way scientists study mice. For example, groups of people could be placed on various experimental, life-extension regimens. When everyone had died, the data could be evaluated, comparing the results with the population at large (the controls). This is known facetiously among some life-extension scientists as "the last person standing" approach. Such a study would be immensely expensive, impractical, and useless to most of us because we would have died long before any results were obtained.

An alternative is to develop a means to measure biological age, to determine how old a person is biologically instead of chronologically. These measurements would be repeated periodically and provide objective determination over relatively short periods of time (six months to several years) whether an individual's life-extension regimen is working or not. An effective program would be reflected by a life-extensionist having a more youthful biological age than his or her chronological peers not following a similar program.

Biological age can be determined by combining various physiological, biochemical, psychological, and anthropometric (or human measurement) parameters that have been found to have a close correlation with chronological age. A variety of these parameters (individually known as biomarkers) can be combined into a battery of tests from which an estimate of biological age can be calculated.

Many functions of the human body cannot be assessed with standard laboratory tests. A large number of testing batteries to measure aging and general health, however, have been designed by many research centers around the world. Numerous equations have been devised to calculate biological age. Although the concept of longitudinal testing has clearly been demonstrated to be of practical value, problems remain.

There is a problem of standardization. There is no single testing battery that has been frequently used to measure biological age in repeated, longitudinal studies. Each research team keeps changing their battery, adding or deleting tests. Also, each team appears bent on making their test batteries as difficult or inconvenient as possible for other scientists to perform. They usually include one or more "esoteric" test that only their research team knows how to conduct.

USEFUL TEST FEATURES

- Standardized
- Convenient and easy to perform routinely
- Inexpensive
- Noninvasive, requiring no more than a blood sample
- Correlated with chronological age
- Preventive
- Measures several levels of aging

To be useful to most life extension practitioners, tests must be easy to perform and noninvasive. They should correlate with chronological age, be preventive in nature, be inexpensive and convenient to use. Ideally, the tests should include parameters that evaluate aging on several levels (i.e., molecular, cellular, organ system, and total body). The tests should evaluate aging based on predictions of the various theories of aging. Biomarkers in this last category may ultimately be the most valuable. They are likely to be most closely associated with (and thus, most accurately reflect) the progress of the aging process.

The goal of life extension is to maintain and, if possible, restore as many biomarkers as possible to an optimum level—i.e., the level of a fit and healthy twenty year old. If it were possible for a 60-year-old person to maintain *all* key biomarkers at that youthful level, that person would, in essence, have a biological age of 20. Their life expectancy, for all practical purposes, would be indefinite. Unfortunately, the life-extension sciences have not advanced to that state yet—but that is the goal.

In the meantime, aging measurements based on a comprehensive panel of biomarkers enable researchers to identify the "weak links" in the human aging process. This knowledge can direct our intervention efforts, and provide us with the best information currently available to evaluate therapeutic regimens and agents. Objective means for evaluating general health, along with the effectiveness of diet, nutritional supplements and their proper dosages and absorption rate, and organ functionality are also important information to determine the right course of action to provide life to one's years.

AGING MEASUREMENT AND BIOMARKER TESTS

According to researcher Ward Dean, M.D., three levels of test batteries should be utilized, since each level is designed for a slightly different purpose.

THREE LEVELS OF TESTS

- *Home testing* —A test battery that could be conducted at home, with a minimum of inexpensive, easily obtainable equipment.
- *Routine office testing* —A routine battery for the physician's office.
- *High end or research battery* —Tests that require equipment not available in most physician's offices, specialized technical expertise, and are fairly expensive.

HOME TESTING

A home-test battery allows life-extensionists who may be on a limited budget to conduct their own measurements. It also enables tests to be performed as frequently as desired. Examples of tests that may be included in the home battery are maximal oxygen uptake field test, oral glucose tolerance test, systolic blood pressure, near vision, static balance, and handgrip strength.

Maximal Oxygen Uptake (VO₂ max) Field Test

VO_2 max measures the oxygen consumed during prolonged exercise. It is an international reference standard for physical fitness. The most accurate values are obtained by direct measurement using a treadmill and physiological monitoring system. A more simple "field test," however, gives remarkably accurate and reproducible results.

This test is performed by determining the time it takes to walk or jog 1-1 ¹/₂ miles. The best place to do this test is on a track. Time how long it takes you to walk or jog 1-1 ¹/₂ miles. Using Figure 8.1 below, find your maximum oxygen uptake. Plot that measure on the Generic Graph (Figure 8.8 on page 147) according to your chronological age.

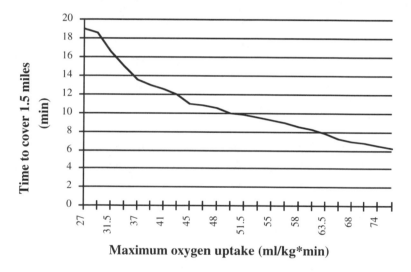

Figure 8.1 Field Test for Measurement of VO₂ max

Data from this chart adapted by Ward Dean, MD from *Biological Aging Measurement.*

If your maximum oxygen uptake increases over time because of your diet, physical-exercise program, or the other applications of your life-extension program, you can say that you have improved the metabolic vitality of virtually all systems. To the extent that this parameter stays the same over time, you can say that aspect of your aging has slowed.

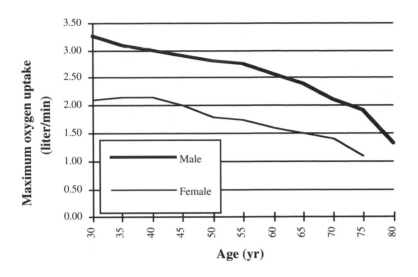

Figure 8.2 Maximal Oxygen Uptake for Men & Women
M. M. Dehn and Bruce, R.A. & K. L. Andersen

Oral Glucose Tolerance Test

The ability of the body to utilize glucose declines progressively with age. This is reflected by a predictable increase in blood glucose one hour after consuming a standard glucose load. To perform this test at home, purchase a simple instrument called a glucometer at any drug store. Instructions are included with the glucometer. It requires only a drop or two of blood, obtained from a "finger stick."

To perform the test, first measure "fasting" blood sugar in the morning before eating or drinking anything except water. Then drink a small can of grape juice, which contains approximately fifty grams of glucose. Exactly one hour later, measure your blood sugar again.

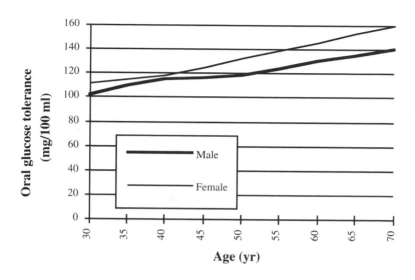

Figure 8.3 Glucose
D. Gillibrand

Systolic Blood Pressure

Hypertension, or high blood pressure, refers to the elevation of blood pressure caused by the malfunctioning of one or more organs that typically maintain normal blood pressure. Diastolic blood pressure, as the heart dilates and fills with blood, does not usually change over time. That parameter generally remains within normal limits throughout the life span. Systolic blood pressure, as the heart contracts and pumps the blood out, often becomes elevated with age. High systolic blood pressure is associated with the increasing hardening of the arterial blood vessels, the heart pumping excess blood, the kidneys excreting too much blood, or a high level of hormones capable of increasing blood pressure. The effects of hypertension are extremely dangerous, since consequences include enlargement and subsequent weakening of the heart muscle, arteriosclerosis, and organ damage or failure. Accurate diagnosis and treatment of high blood pressure is essential.

Drug stores sell blood pressure cuffs and stethoscopes. Blood pressure can be easily measured at home. Home readings actually may be more accurate than readings in a doctor's office, since artificial elevation may occur due to anxiety by being in a doctor's office. Follow the instructions that come with the instrument and graph your data chronologically. In the next graph, the general rise in systolic pressure reflects average aging.

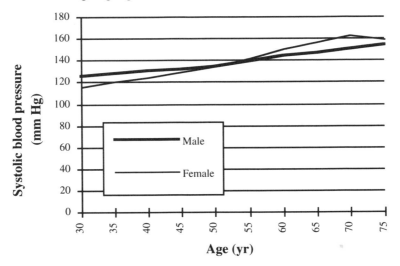

Figure 8.4 Systolic Blood Pressure

Framingham Study

Near Vision

The lens of the eye becomes progressively less elastic resulting in "old age sight" (presbyopia) as aging occurs. People usually notice this in their early forties. To test for near vision, you need a yardstick marked in centimeters and a business card. If you normally wear glasses or contact lenses for distance vision, wear them when conducting this test.

Hold one end of the yardstick against the cheekbone below the eye being tested. With the other hand, hold the business card at a distance where it can be comfortably read. Slowly bring it closer to the eye, until it begins to become blurry. Using the yardstick, measure the closest distance (in centimeters) at which the small print is in sharp focus. Chart your data on the Generic Graph on page 147.

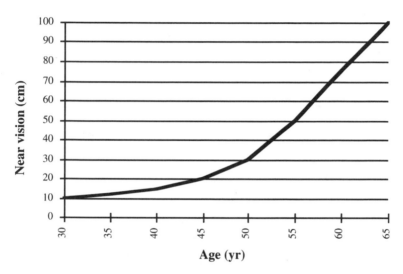

Figure 8.5 Near Vision

The area represents the distance at which 90 percent of the population can see near objects clearly.

R.F. Morgan and J. Wilson; A. Duane, and R. Sekuler

Static Balance

Researchers generally believe that the more integrated the function, the more sensitive it is to the aging process. Testing static balance demonstrates the overall neuromuscular functioning of your body.

To perform this test, stand unsupported on your left leg (if you are right-handed), hands on hips with eyes closed. Time the number of seconds you are able to do this. Repeat the test three times at five-minute intervals. Your score is the longest duration in seconds that you can stand without loss of balance. Chart your score on the Generic Graph (page 147).

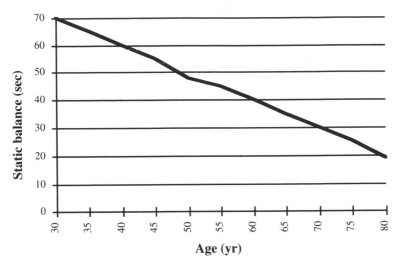

Figure 8.6 Static Balance Test on One Leg
H. Shimokata

Handgrip Strength

Handgrip strength is one of the oldest tests used to measure aging. It reflects both neurologic function and muscular vitality in terms of mass and strength. It is measured with a handgrip dynamometer.

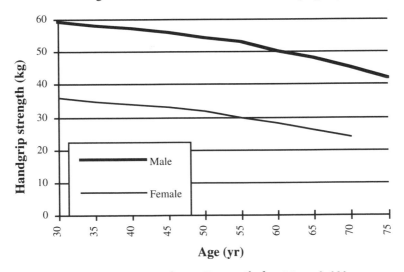

Figure 8.7 Handgrip Strength for Men & Women
A. Damon et al.

Generic Graph

The graph below can be used to chart the scores from any of the tests we've discussed thus far. Make as many copies as you need; enlarge if necessary. Be sure to write in the test name, the dates, the normal reference range, and the units of measurement, as well as the observed results. Use a separate graph for each different variable you are tracking. As you test yourself several times in the future, you plot your data on the graph for that test. Then you can compare your scores to evaluate if you are making progress in your life-extension program.

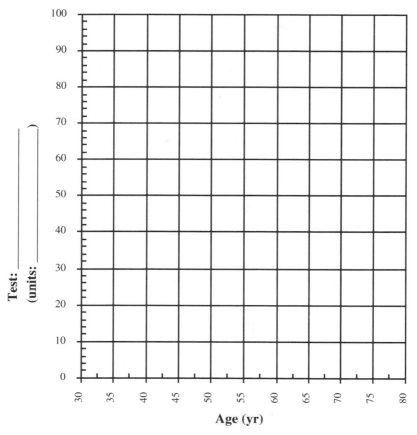

Figure 8.8 Generic Graph

ROUTINE OFFICE TESTING

Routine office tests are more sophisticated than the ones performed at home. They require a clinical laboratory, specialized equipment, or skills that only health-care personnel are likely to possess. Most physicians who perform routine physical examinations have access to the equipment required for these tests. Recommendations for tests to be included in the routine office-test battery include examination of hair, urine, saliva, blood, and audiovisual acuity. You can use the generic graphs to plot your scores from these tests over time. Use the values supplied by the laboratory. Standardized values are provided in the following discussion which you can use if none are available from the laboratory. Life extensionists recommend that you use the results achieved by 20 year olds as a reference.

Hair Analysis

Hair analysis is a straightforward technique for analyzing the levels of nutritional minerals and toxic metals in a person's body. It is a standard method of analysis in nutritional medicine and toxicology.

Blood and urine analyses show only what has been present in the body in the most recent past. Hair, on the other hand, grows slowly and is a very stable protein. It accumulates elements from the blood stream over a long period of time. Hair analysis shows the body's general nutritional status and level of exposure to certain toxins. A standard panel of analyses would include the elements in Table 8.9.

A convenient and cost-effective technique, hair analysis is an essential tool in a scientific approach to personal nutrition. It is a noninvasive procedure. Hair may be stored nearly indefinitely, and hair may be easily mailed to a diagnostic laboratory with no requirements for special handling.

TABLE 8.9 ELEMENTS OFTEN FOUND IN HAIR

Nutritional Minerals		Toxic Metals
Calcium	Manganese	Lead
Magnesium	Cobalt	Mercury
Zinc	Iron	Calcium
Copper	Lithium	Arsenic
Chromium	Molybdenum	Nickel
Sodium	Phosphorous	Aluminum
Potassium	Vanadium	
Selenium	Germanium	

Hair analysis is important to life-extensionists for two reasons. First, you have high levels of toxic metals in your body, you would want to lower your exposure, and if necessary, do displacement therapy. Displacement therapy consists of drugs, supplements, or a diet that removes toxins from your body. Second, your nutritional mineral analysis may indicate a need to increase or decrease intake of nutritional minerals with foods or with supplements. Instructions for how to evaluate your results usually accompany each analysis.

There are theoretical benefits from using hair analysis as a tool in aging intervention. Dr. William H. Strain of the Case Western Reserve University School of Medicine in Cleveland, Ohio, believes that hair analysis offers potential for study and control of the aging process. In an abstract published in *AGE*, the journal of the American Aging Association, Strain reported that up to sixty elements may be readily determined in hair by atomic-absorption spectroscopy, or by a more elaborate technique known as ICP arc spectroscopy. He noted that data from several thousand analyses have indicated that many trace-element deficiencies develop with aging. Many of these deficiencies may be corrected by dietary modifications. Age-adjusted values for most elements demonstrated to be of clinical significance have recently been determined by researchers Gordon, Schauss and Jackson. Dr. Strain believes that improved analytical capabilities offer the dramatic potential to identify trace-mineral deficiencies or toxicities, restore tissue mineral levels to optimum, and possibly eventually slow the aging process.

DNA Damage Assessment

There is a urine test developed by University of California at Berkeley's Professor Bruce Ames. It is an assay of thymine glycol, which determines the amount of DNA damage occurring in an individual.

Serum Cholesterol

Serum cholesterol tends to increase in both males and females with increase in age. Elevated cholesterol level is associated with coronary artery disease. The prevailing opinion about amounts and percentages of cholesterol that are harmful seems to keep changing. In general, if your cholesterol remains under 180 mg/dl, it is presumed that your risk of heart attack from atherosclerosis is minimal and that you may not need to measure the high-density lipoprotein level. If, however, your cholesterol is over 220, then the total cholesterol/HDL ratio becomes important.

In stages of life before arterial calcification occurs, total cholesterol is amenable to control by diet and exercise. The optimal reference range for males and females is 125 to 175 mg/dl.

HDL Cholesterol

High density lipoprotein (HDL) is a component of the total cholesterol. The higher the amount of HDL cholesterol in relationship to the total cholesterol the better. The absolute value of HDL by itself usually does not mean much. If you wish to graph your HDL, use the current reference ranges from your laboratory report.

Fibrinogen

Fibrinogen is a high-molecular-weight blood protein involved in blood coagulation. Fibrinogen is converted to fibrin through the action of thrombin. Fibrinogen increases with age, and contributes to the increased risk of thromboembolic disease, or blood clots, in the elderly. The optimal reference range for males and females is 160 to 220 mg/dl.

Creatinine Clearance

Creatinine clearance, or removal of protein from the blood by the kidney, declines with age. This reflects the loss of nephrons in the kidney, and atherosclerosis of renal arteries. The optimal reference range for males and females is 110 to 180 mL/min/1.73 m²

Luteinizing Hormone

Luteinizing hormone (LH) rises with age, due to inadequate suppression by decreased sex-hormone secretion. The optimum reference range for males is 1 to 2.5 mI.U./mL and for females 3 to 4.5 mI.U./mL.

Follicle Stimulating Hormone

Follicle stimulating hormone (FSH) also rises with age, also due to inadequate suppression by decreased sex-hormone secretion. The optimal range for males is .5 to 4 mI.U./mL and for females, 1 to 20 mI.U./mL.

Free Testosterone

Free testosterone in males declines with age, due to a combination of decreased output and increased testosterone-binding globulin. Optimal range is 4.5 to 11 mg/mL.

Estradiol

Estradiol decreases with age in women, but *increases* in men. The optimal range for males is 85 to 125 pmol/L and for females, 400 to 510 pmol/L.

Tri-iodothyronine

Tri-iodothyronine (T3) declines with age, partially reflecting a breakdown in the "energy homeostat." Optimal range for males and females is 115 to 140 mg/dl.

Thyroid Stimulating Hormone

Thyroid stimulating hormone (TSH) increases slightly with age, mostly after age 50. TSH is also related to breakdown in the "energy homeostat." Optimal range for both males and females is 0 to 4.

Adrenal Stress Index

The adrenal stress index (ASI) measures the daily fluctuations of salivary free cortisol, and correlates them with salivary dehydroepiandrosterone-sulfate (DHEA-S). This graphical correlation allows the determination of normal, adapted, and maladapted stress-response patterns. This innovative test is totally noninvasive, requiring only four timed salivary specimens.

Forced Vital Capacity

Forced vital capacity (FVC) declines progressively and predictably with age. Although the cause is unknown, it is believed to be due to age-related muscle weakness and other changes in the chest wall. Many investigators label FVC as the best predictor of subsequent longevity. If you have this test done, use the values for 20-year-old normals for your height and sex.

Near and Distance Visual Acuities

Vision, our most important sense, also unfortunately declines with age. Obtain your data from your routine ophthalmologic examination, using 20/20 as the optimal value.

Audiometry

Hearing is the most important sense next to vision. Hearing loss in decibels is measured at many different frequencies. To use this test to measure aging, average the decibel values (or volume you are able to hear) between 3000 and 6000 c.p.s. or Hz. Chart the values for the right and left ears on separate graphs. The loss of hearing acuity with age is thought to be due to destruction of the tiny hair cells in the inner ear.

"HIGH END" OR RESEARCH BATTERY

Tests in the research battery include more expensive tests, or esoteric tests that require expensive equipment or skills not generally available in physicians' offices.

Dehydroepiandrosterone-sulfate

Next to cholesterol, dehydroepiandrosterone-sulfate (DHEA–S) is the most abundant steroid (fat-soluble hormone) in the body. It declines rapidly with age, and may be one of the most significant biomarkers. Low DHEA levels are correlated with increased incidence of a number of diseases in addition to old age. However, oral supplementation of DHEA does not seem to increase maximum life span.

Melatonin

Melatonin is the hormone produced by the pineal gland. The pineal gland appears to be a "master gland," controlling the sleep-wake cycle and other daily rhythms. Melatonin levels generally begin rising in the evening, peaking one to two hours after sleep. With increasing age, however, peak melatonin levels progressively decrease and occur *later* in the evening.

Because peak melatonin levels occur at night, blood sampling must be performed between midnight and three a.m. Few physicians' offices remain open at this time and the values would likely be skewed, since the subject would have to remain awake, suppressing melatonin levels. Consequently, this test should be conducted in a hospital or research facility. Melatonin supplements are becoming popular and hold promise of extending life and youthfulness, or at least getting a good night's sleep, which always benefits the body.

Maximal Oxygen Uptake

In the office or research facility this test is conducted using a treadmill and physiological monitoring device. The device accurately measures the volume and concentration of expired gases. It is an international reference standard for physical fitness.

Basal Metabolic Rate

The basal metabolic rate is best measured with a whole-body calorimeter, suitable for use in a physician's office. The calorimeter, designed by Dr. Daniel Hershey, accurately determines the basal metabolic rate. It also provides a person's minimal caloric requirement, used by many weight-loss clinics to assist with diet planning. In addition, it yields a prediction of *future remaining life span.*

Serum Lipid Peroxide Levels

In accordance with the free-radical theory of aging, damaging lipid peroxides increase with age. Yagi developed a simple and reliable method to determine the lipid peroxide level in human blood.

Cross-Linking Index

A serum assay that measures the degree of intermolecular cross-linking has been developed. This test has been primarily designed to evaluate the progression of osteoporosis. No age-related values have yet been determined. It appears to offer promise as a biomarker to evaluate Bjorksten's cross-linkage theory of aging.

Essential Metabolic Analysis™

Until recently, it was difficult to accurately assess a person's nutrient status. Routine blood tests of serum vitamin levels measure only the vitamin levels at the instant the blood was drawn. These levels do not correspond to levels or functions of nutrients inside cells. Blood tests do not assess whether the amount of a particular nutrient is adequate or inadequate for a particular individual. A quantitative determination of long-term levels of nutrients within cells and tissues, and an evaluation of their metabolic activity would offer a much deeper insight into nutritional status. The problem has been to develop such a test.

The best way to assess the functional status of an individual is by analyzing living, metabolically active cells that reflect an individual's functional nutritional status. In other words, instead of measuring *how much* nutrient is present, the best way is to measure *how well* a nutrient works.

Dr. William Shive of the University of Texas developed an assay using peripheral lymphocytes to accomplish just such a functional test that is simple and easy for your physician to perform. Peripheral lymphocytes are white blood cells that the body stores in peripheral locations for long periods of time. There are a few reasons why lymphocytes are an excellent choice for such analysis. Lymphocytes are readily available in large numbers in a normal blood sample. They exhibit metabolic pathways common to other cells. In addition, they provide an excellent picture of an individual's time-averaged nutritional status from the previous year.

Dr. Shive developed and patented a special growth medium (CFBI 1000™) that supports optimal growth of human lymphocytes. By removing essential nutrients one at a time from the growth medium, Dr. Shive forced the lymphocytes to rely upon their reserve of that nutrient to support their growth. In this manner, the functional status of most nutrients could be assessed. Subjects whose lymphocytes had growth lower than "normal" ranges after the deletion of a specific nutrient had decreased functional status of that nutrient.

Subjects who had been determined to be deficient in a nutrient were supplemented with that nutrient. When they were later retested, 95 percent of the values of most abnormal nutrient levels either became within normal ranges, or closer to the norm.

EMA™ (essential metabolics analysis) offers a number of advantages over other assays for nutrient status. First and foremost is the concept of measuring cell *function*, instead of measuring quantitative levels of a nutrient. Second, EMA™ offers a deeper insight into each individual's "metabolic machinery" from a nutritional point of view. Other advantages of the EMA™ analysis are a perspective on long-term nutritional status; individualized treatment that is based on clinically and scientifically valid information; and a functional assessment of nutrient levels that are derived from a dynamic rather than a static situation.

Computerized Diet Analysis

Dietary management for nutritional deficiencies and for altering the percentage of fat, carbohydrate, and other dietary constituents is an extremely powerful tool in health and medicine. Further, caloric restriction is the primary technique that has been shown to slow biological aging and extend the maximum life span to a significant degree. Thus, dietary management is an important life-extension and disease-prevention technique. There are two computerized diet analysis systems that are designed specifically with life extension in mind.

PREVENTIVE MEDICINE & LIFE EXTENSION GO HAND IN HAND

The entire field of measuring biomarkers to study aging is rapidly evolving. The results of many of the routine tests in the annual physical can be used as parameters for aging. The home tests can be used to track vitality over time. The data can be used to evaluate risk to certain diseases. Thus, preventive medicine and life extension go hand in hand.

The prudent life-extensionist can have the recommended tests performed at periodic intervals every three to six months. It is important to monitor the trends seen in the result. At a future date, the data can be used to calculate biological ages retroactively, when more advanced equations become available. The goal of life extension is to restore and maintain each parameter at as youthful a level as possible.

CHAPTER NINE

PHASE I LIFE EXTENSION: REDUCING DISEASE

Life-extension applications can be divided into two phases. This distinction may not always be clear in practice, but it is important to understand the theoretical difference. Phase I applications prevent life-shortening disease but do not affect biological aging. Phase II applications prevent life-shortening disease and maintain biological vitality by slowing or reversing biological aging.

PHASE I APPLICATIONS FOR LIFE EXTENSION

A modality can be a drug, a nutrient, a set of procedures that reactivates a genetic program, a mantra or sequence of thoughts, a philosophy or even a social system. Any modality that does not increase the maximum genetic life span but does cause an increase in the average life-expectancy (i.e., 50 percent of those using the therapy survive longer) is called a "Phase I" life-extension application. Stated in another way, Phase I methods prevent death from life-shortening disease but do not affect biological aging. The method enables a person to live to the full extent of his or her genetically, predetermined life span. To demonstrate this point, look at the following comparative survival curves.

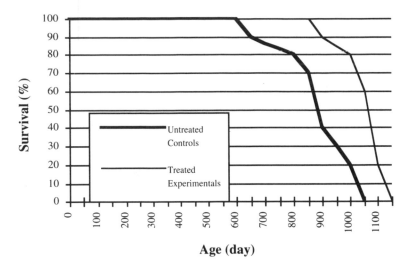

Figure 9.1 Survival Curve for Phase I Life Extension

Data in this chart adapted by Chadd Everone from *Life-Extension Manual.*

ANIMAL STUDIES

Looking at Figure 9.1 we can see that the experimental agent (treated group) enabled more of the animals to live out the full genetic potential of their particular strain. It did not, however, increase the maximum genetic life span. It did not slow aging or cause regeneration. Essentially, this is what has been happening to human populations in advanced industrialized societies over the last several centuries. One by one, the causes of premature death have been brought under control, the average life expectancy has steadily increased to its present extent of approximately seventy years, with more people living into senescence.

HUMAN STUDIES

If the intervention works in animals it will probably work in humans is the basic premise. Definitive studies of life-extension agents can only be done in animals that are genetically well understood. Less definitive studies are controlled clinical experiments with human beings. One such study is the Baltimore Longitudinal Study that studied lifestyle, disease risk, and biomarkers of aging and health. Another is the Framingham Study of cardiovascular disease. A host of other studies deal with specific diseases. These studies use small groups of selected individuals, representative of the human population at large. Subjects are tested on a variety of measures and retested after a long period of time. Generalizations are made about the changes in the various measures.

EPIDEMIOLOGICAL STUDIES

Another approach are the epidemiological studies correlating cause and effect of the disease and health characteristics of large classes of people. Epidemiological studies are less definitive than research on case-selected human groups, which, in turn, are less definitive than well-designed animal studies. The highest degree of certainty is when there occurs a good correlation and consistency of finding between all three types of evidence.

WHAT YOU "DON'T" DO

Among gerontologists, there is a maxim that has circulated for as long as anyone can remember: "Life extension is not so much what you do as it is what you do not do." This statement is certainly valid when it comes to the few practical "don'ts" that when not done are correlated with the most significant life extension.

DON'TS FOR EXTENDING LIFE

- Do not smoke
- Do not overeat
- Do not drink much alcohol
- Do not expose yourself to toxic substances
- Do not lead a sedentary and anxiety-filled life

With a well-regimented program that integrates these common and well-established health practices, the average person could maintain vitality and prevent disease to a significant extent, increasing life expectancy by as much as 20 percent. These practices, however, will make only a modest contribution to slowing biological aging and certainly will not reverse it. Still, ten to twenty additional years of healthy life span should be worth some effort and expense. That might be just long enough to take advantage of big breakthroughs that seem inevitable in the future.

THE APPLICATION OF PHASE I

Well-established practices in Phase I life extension in animal studies, in selected groups of humans, and in epidemiological studies include the following categories:

TOXICOLOGY

Life expectancy can be extended and risk to disease lowered by the avoidance of excessive exposure to toxic substances. Toxic substances include tobacco, alcohol, and drugs—both therapeutic and recreational drugs. Natural toxins include allergenic and infectious agents. Finally, there are industrial chemicals, fumes, industrial dust, and toxins in many household products and in some of the foods we eat.

NUTRITION

To a substantial degree, life expectancy can be extended and risk to disease lowered by maintaining a well-balanced diet. A well-balanced diet is one low in fat and protein, and high in complex carbohydrates and fiber, which reduces the risk of obesity. Supplementation of a full-spectrum vitamin and mineral compound that includes antioxidant properties can buffer periodic dietary inadequacies and metabolic stress.

PHYSICAL EXERCISE

Life expectancy can be extended and risk to disease lowered by routine and appropriate exercises in which muscle tissue is strengthened, the cardiovascular system is conditioned, and flexibility is enhanced.

PREVENTIVE AND CURATIVE MEDICINE

Health restoration in the form of diet, exercise, relaxation, chiropractic, massage, or any one of a number of "natural" therapies can cure disease and thereby extend life. Obviously, if disease can be prevented, that will make a major contribution to fulfilling genetic potential in a state of optimal health. The same is true with utilizing good medical management if a disease does occur. Unless necessary, aggressive medical treatment is generally avoided in the phase I approach.

PSYCHOLOGICAL ASPECTS

In a very fundamental way, life extension is a philosophical and psychological enterprise. Attitude and mind-set are prerequisite to implementing the recommendations for a life-extension type of lifestyle, and an active social and intellectual life seem to carry one a long way.

BASIC CONCEPTS OF PHASE I

There are numerous sources of information on well-established health practices and as many ways of implementing these practices as there are individuals who take this path. Most Phase I practices are already well known by people who are interested in health. It is worthwhile, however, to review these basic concepts of Phase I application.

TOXICOLOGY

Any substance that your body needs or can use to maintain its natural functions and that is supplied by an outside source is, by definition, a nutrient. Anything other than a nutrient is likely to be a toxin.

You breathe in, ingest, touch, harbor in your intestine, and otherwise take into your body all kinds of foreign substances that damage cells and interfere with metabolic processes. In high amounts, such toxins can cause disease, diminish health and vitality, and shorten the natural life span. However, even when animals are raised in a completely sterile and toxin-free environment, only the average life span is increased. Only a minimal increment can be seen on maximum life span. In other words, even though you are constantly being bombarded by a massive array of toxins, you intrinsically have sufficient repair and protective mechanisms so that a modest level of exposure does not impact much on health.

Air pollution and water pollution are obvious sources of exposure to toxic substances. What is not so obvious is that natural substances, often found in the food you eat, are a major source of toxins.

Bruce Ames' Surprising Discoveries

Toxicology, cancer, aging, environmental issues and politics all intertwine in the career of scientist Bruce Ames, Professor of Biochemistry at the University of California, Berkeley. Profiling his work over the years will illustrate some important developments.

During the early 1960s, Ames did extensive research on toxicity of industrial chemicals and their carcinogenic potential. He gained wide notoriety for sounding the alarm that industry was introducing thousands of new chemicals into the environment without much, if any, research on their toxic effects. The Zeitgeist or popular spirit of the times was anti-establishment and anti-industry. The environmental and health movements eagerly used his pronouncements in support of their causes. Testing the toxicity of a single chemical requires thousands of animals exposed to graduated doses, over a period of time, with meticulous record keeping and observation. This is a laborious, time-consuming, and expensive routine, which industry is not inclined to do and government is reticent to impose. Because of these barriers, Ames began genetically engineering a single-cell model, using the bacterium salmonella typhimurium. This bacterium was used to test the mu-tagenic and carcinogenic effects of chemicals and enables the mass screening of the effects in a short period of time, at minimal cost. This method is known as the Ames Mutagenicity Test and is widely used today.

During the years that followed the development of his mutagenic-ity test, Ames proceeded to evaluate hundreds of industrial chemicals, publishing his findings as he went. His laboratory was a veritable factory for testing insecticides, herbicides, epoxy compounds—the entire port-folio of the multinational petrochemical industry. In 1975, he found hair dyes to be mutagenic, warning that some 20 million women, many of child-bearing age, were being exposed to carcinogens. In 1977, he reported that the flame-retardant chemical that was being added to children's sleepwear was a possible cancer hazard that was absorbed through the skin. Also that year, he reported that certain chemothera-peutic agents for cancer were mutagenic and therefore possibly cancer causing.

Although a piranha to established commercial interests, Ames has remained beyond reproach because his science has been of the highest caliber. It was his continued pursuit of the science that eventually surprised everyone, both his political opponents and his supporters. In 1979 Ames announced that he had been testing the mutagenicity of constituents of natural foods, mostly plant foods, and was finding them to be highly toxic also. This, he pointed out, should not be surprising because plants, unlike animals, do not have active immune systems mediated by special types of cells. Plants have passive immune systems that depend on their ability to produce toxic substances. These toxic substances protect plants from bacteria, fungi, insects and animals that feed on them. Ames labeled these "natural pesticides."

It might be that one of the reasons why caloric restriction has such a beneficial biological effect is due to reduced exposure to natural carcinogens in food. Carcinogens induce cancer by damaging DNA directly or indirectly, with one of the mechanisms being free-radical reactions. There is evidence that antioxidant defenses prevent cancer and that supplemental antioxidants lower the risk to cancer. As an assessment of aging and risk to cancer, Ames has devised a urine test–an assay of thymine glycol–to determine the amount of DNA damage occurring in an individual. His current line of investigations continue in this area.

NATURAL PESTICIDE POISONING

Results indicate that, when viewed against the large background of naturally occurring carcinogens in typical portions of common foods, the residues of synthetic pesticides or environmental pollutants rank low. . .99.99% (by weight) of the pesticides in the American diet are chemicals that plants produce to defend themselves. . .carcinogenic hazards from current levels of pesticide residues or water pollution are likely to be of minimal concern relative to the background levels of natural substances, though one cannot say whether these natural exposures are likely to be of major or minor importance.

—Bruce Ames

To summarize, the toxicology approach to life extension is to minimize exposure to toxic substances. On a practical level this means not to smoke or work in an environment where others do. Make sure that household chemicals are sealed to prevent outgassing. When you use solvents, glues and other toxins, make sure you are in a well-ventilated area. If you work in an industrial environment in which there is dust and assorted chemicals, wear a mask in appropriate situations and exert pressure on management to keep the surroundings cleaned and well ventilated. If you have asthma or allergies, consult a medical professional about how to investigate and manage your environment. Use a carbon filter for drinking water.

The general air quality in your geographical area is a political issue to be approached through government agencies. Alternatively you can move to an area of cleaner air. Maintain a diet high in fresh fruits and vegetables and supplement your nutrition with appropriate antioxidants.

NUTRITION

The nutritional approach to living a long and disease free life is eating a well-balanced diet and restricting caloric intake. The main issue becomes how to reorganize behavior and lifestyle so that food intake is minimized. The specific plan will vary by individual.

If you cannot restrict total calories, then what you eat becomes an important issue. Although there is a great deal of research being done in nutrition, as it relates to disease and health, the main recommendations are simple and well-established from studies in animals, selected human populations, and epidemiology.

Excessive dietary fat, which is fat intake greater that 20% of total calories, increases a person's risk of contracting cancer and heart disease. Increased fiber in the diet provides bulk without calories, absorbs some of the fat so that it is not digested and assimilated, and lowers mutagenic agents that are generated by normal bacteria in the bowel. Consequently, a low-fat diet with high-fiber foods like vegetables, grains, legumes, and fruits is recommended. This should lower the risk of stroke, heart disease, and cancer, which accounts for 80% of premature deaths.

PHYSICAL EXERCISE

The late Linus Pauling contributed much to science during the 20th century. His research in the 1930s advanced the understanding of molecular structures. For that work, he received the Nobel Prize in 1954. In the mid-1950s, Pauling almost beat Watson and Crick in describing the structure of DNA. In the 1960s, he began his work in orthomolecular medicine which included the use of natural molecules for therapeutic applications. He became a major proponent for the use of vitamin C and nutrition for health and treatment of disease.

Pauling's interest ranged far and wide. In 1987, at a conference on gerontology, he gave a presentation on a variety of applications that he thought would be useful for life extension. Afterward, during the question-and-answer period, it was asked why he had not mentioned physical exercise as an important modality. Pauling replied that he had reviewed extensively the scientific research on exercise and had come to the conclusion that any additional length in life span that might be gained by exercising was less than the amount of time it took to do the exercising! Therefore he preferred to spend his time thinking and talking rather than straining.

It seems obvious that physical exercise would improve the quality of life and also improve the length or quantity of life. However, both criteria, quality and quantity, are still contested. Pauling lived for over 90 years, probably without any serious physical exercise after age 40. He was active and productive for virtually his entire life span. On the other hand, in 1993, investigators at the University of Helsinki in Finland reviewed the life span of a large number of world-class male athletes, and reported that they had increased life expectancy due to a decrease in cardiovascular mortality. But as far as maximum life span vwas conerned, no increase was found. In fact, the average high-performance athlete had a life span of about seventy-eight years, which although above average, is still almost two decades less than Pauling's life span.

In some controlled animal experiments, average life expectancy was increased by exercise. In other such experiments, exercise was correlated with a somewhat decrease in average life expectancy. Even in the area of the prevention of cardiovascular disease, often a lean, middle-aged world-class runner dies suddenly from a heart attack. Recent reports indicate a significant decrease in breast cancer in women who exercise three times a week for forty-five minutes or more. Breast cancer is highly influenced by female hormones, and some experts speculate that the decreased tumor incidence might be due to an exercise-induced suppression of these hormones.

It is commonly assumed that exercise helps to control appetite and thus would be useful in the reinforcement of caloric restriction. However, some studies reveal an increase in appetite with exercise.

Physical exercise is probably a matter of personal aesthetics. A reasonably well-conditioned body looks better and performs better. If done properly, exercise probably contributes to the prevention of heart attack, stroke, cancer, osteoporosis, arthritis, and other chronic diseases. In addition, exercise elevates endorphins, which can be euphoric, and induces relaxation which overcomes the negative effects of anxiety.

A proper exercise regimen has three main objectives: cardiovascular conditioning, muscle strengthening, and flexibility. A good workout program is usually four to eight hours per week. If you can involve friends and members of your family, exercising can be a good medium of social interaction.

For cardiovascular conditioning, the standard protocol is any activity such as walking, jogging, swimming, or other movement that involves the large muscles and cause the heart rate to increase. Three times a week, exercise aerobically (i.e., not out of breath) for a sustained period of about thirty to forty-five minutes. Start out slowly and build your endurance capacity.

For muscle strengthening, weight-resistance exercise three times a week using free weights or Nautilus-type machines is the norm. Initially, it is advised to follow the instructions of a trainer. Increase the level of resistance at a pace that is comfortable for you personally.

For flexibility, a trainer in a weight room can usually recommend a satisfactory set of stretching postures. Alternatively, yoga, tai chi and other physical meditation techniques can keep one supple and spry as one ages.

PREVENTIVE AND CURATIVE MEDICINE

The above-recommended procedures in toxicology, nutrition, and physical conditioning should make a large contribution to improving and maintaining general health and preventing medical problems. In addition, periodic multiphasic examinations that include a hands-on physical and review of your biological systems by a physician, comprehensive blood chemistries and cell counts, exercise electrocardiography, and any other tests like aging biomarkers is advised. Ask your physician for an evaluation of your personal risk profile. Also, look for any subclinical disorders and seek appropriate measures of intervention.

If you do have a medical problem, do not rush into therapy unless it is really necessary. Get a clear idea about the different prognoses for different therapies and compare it to a prognosis for no therapy. Ask your physician about what is called an "observational" approach, in which the disease process is monitored closely, during which time you aggressively implement a program of dietary modification, exercise, massage, and any health technique that might be advisable. Seek second and third opinions about the diagnosis and therapeutic strategy. Do research to seek what is considered state-of-the-art therapy. Some diseases render themselves to medical treatments that are highly efficacious and do not have significant side effects. Others diseases do not. Think of your physician as being a technical consultant, with you assuming as much of the responsibility as possible for managing your own health problem.

PSYCHOLOGICAL ASPECTS

People say a positive attitude contributes to a long and productive life, and being happy is beneficial in overcoming disease. Yet nihilists, pessimists, and people who have little sense of humor seem to live as long and sometimes even more productive a life as others. Besides, even if it were true that such positive psychology were beneficial, how would it be possible to create such positiveness if a person did not already have it by nature? This is a realm that everyone agrees is important yet there are no objective criteria.

Certainly, human beings are social animals. Intellectual curiosity and involvement give more meaning to life and make a person more vital. But visit any geriatric facility and you will witness large numbers of people living a long time without much mental stimulation. The body seems to hang on as long as it can even if the person is not happy, not stimulated, or not even there mentally.

Rather than speculate about what psychological attributes might contribute to life extension, it is probably more productive to look at the inverse proposition. Given physical life extension, what psychological attributes might be appropriate to that situation?

Having a life-extension attitude puts more of the responsibility for managing your own personal existential dilemma on to you. Perhaps in anticipation of a relatively short life span, a person can put up with mediocrity and misery more easily, as it is futile to try and it will all end soon. But in the life-extension scenario, whatever you have made of your life will continue even longer unless you make changes. If you are dissatisfied with your life, that will continue or even worsen unless you make the improvements. If you have made accomplishments and are satisfied with your life, you will probably find that you must nurture and enhance your investments, otherwise they atrophy.

The slogan "Think globally act locally" takes on more tangible meaning. You must plan and act on your survival contingencies over a longer period of time and within a broader more global perspective. For example, if in thirty to fifty years, the fossil fuel reserves become depleted as many experts predict, where do you place yourself geographically to mitigate the negative impact on you? Further, how might you benefit from the massive industrial retooling that will have to take place to adapt to a civilization without fossil fuel? There are big opportunities in big transitions.

Life extension is already happening with or without conscious design or a large-scale concerted scientific effort. The three-stage life cycle of thirty years for development and acculturation, to thirty-five years of production, to short-term retirement before death is obsolete in advanced societies. Virtually all social institutions that reinforced that paradigm are disintegrating.

Start thinking about your existence from the life-extension perspective. Given forty to fifty years in front of you, what do you want to be, or, rather, *who do you want to be?* Where do you want to be? With whom do you want to be? Instead of looking for the meaning of life, first consider what meaning you want to give to your life. If you follow this line of thought, you will probably find that a wide spectrum of potentialities open and you can get on with the business of being born.

CHAPTER TEN

PHASE II LIFE EXTENSION: EXTENDING LIFE SPAN

A modality such as a drug, a nutrient, a set of procedures that reactivates a genetic program that causes a shift of the normal survival curve to increase both the survival of the fiftieth percentile and the maximum, genetic life span is called a Phase II life-extension application. In other words, the modality prevents life-shortening disease and maintains biological vitality by means of slowing or reversing one or more aspects of biological aging, or both.

Out of the thousands of experiments that have been performed, caloric restriction is one modality that has shown strong evidence to extend maximum life span. Over the years experiments have been done with vitamins, minerals, amino acids, fish oils, and different distributions of protein, fat, and carbohydrates in the diet, but none have consistently shown the promise caloric restriction presents.

Scientists have experimented with a technique called *parabiosis*, in which the blood stream of an old animal is connected to that of a young animal. The objective was to discover a hormone or metabolic factor operative in the young and not in the old. The factor was not found, and the technique did not increase maximum life span. Research was conducted on testosterone, estrogen, thyroid, adrenal, and a host of other hormones without significant Phase II results. It is true that supplements of certain biochemicals such as melatonin, deprenyl, pineal polypeptide extract, and Dilantin have been shown to extend maximum life span. Yet research has shown that the primary technique that can extend maximum genetic life span is caloric restriction.

The survival curve below demonstrates a Phase II life-extension application.

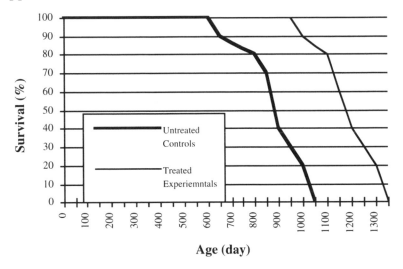

Figure 10.1 Survival Curve for Phase II Life Extension

Data in this chart adapted by Chadd Everone from *Life-Extension Manual.*

CALORIC RESTRICTION

Walford explains the practical applications of caloric restriction to the human life span from his work on animal experiments and from his own personal experience. More recently his work in the Biosphere 2 has yielded fascinating results. The Biosphere 2 was an experiment in which eight people (four men and four women) lived in a sealed, ecologically self-sustaining dome in the Arizona desert for a period of two years, ending in 1993. In part the experiment was to see if people could sustain themselves solely on food they grew. The "Biospherians" demonstrated that they could grow enough food to feed themselves on a diet of about 1,800 calories per day per person. And by accident the first real controlled caloric-restriction experiment with humans was performed.

The restricted diet of the Biospherians was different from the diets Walford used in experimental animals. The essential difference was that a highly synthetic diet was given to the animals and a completely natural diet to the people in Biosphere 2.

Recall in a previous section on caloric restriction that the greatest extension of life span both mean and maximum life was obtained on what would be considered the extreme in synthetic diets. The animal diet consisted of a pelletized feed of 26% crude protein, 4% lard, 49% sugar, 15% starch, and synthesized vitamins and minerals. A synthetic diet might have other benefits. For example, metabolic energy is devoted to breaking down natural foods into their elemental units. In a synthetic diet much of this breakdown has already been accomplished by the refining process. Thus, a synthetic diet theoretically reduces wear and tear by requiring less metabolic work to gain adequate nutrition. Further, plant foods (fruits, grains, and vegetables) protect themselves from insects, fungi, and bacteria by means of naturally produced potent toxic chemicals. Eating a diet high in plant material means ingesting a massive load of toxins. These toxins are reduced to a minimum in a synthetic diet.

In contrast with the synthetic animal diets used in his experiments, Walford recommends a diet for humans based on plant foods. His central idea is that foods high in fiber, but with little caloric value (leafy greens, sprouts, celery), and high in starch (predominantly bananas, beets, potatoes), yield a diet low in caloric value but dense in all other essential nutrients and one that also satisfies appetite.

There are hundreds of different diet programs, each claiming some unique benefit. For life-extension purposes, however, the essential concept is low total calories with adequate amounts of other essential nutrients. You may use a number of strategies to achieve this. You can fast every third day. You can have only two meals per day. You can have five very small meals per day. You can feast one day per week and be tightly restricted the other six. According to Walford's work the benefits are derived by eating an average of about 1,800 calories daily. This average, however, can be spread over a fairly long period of time.

In all restricted diets, supplementing with a full-spectrum vitamin and mineral compound may be a good idea, depending on which substances are not readily provided in the food. There are normal and routine precautions when going on any restricted diet. If you are under medical treatment, ask your physician if there are any contra-indications with your condition. Do not lose weight rapidly (two or three pounds per week is fine). If you experience any dizziness or unusual symptoms, retreat from the diet and consult your physician. The physical objective of the restricted diet is to achieve a body weight that is close to what you had at about the age of twenty or, better, a body fat percentage of 10–15 percent for men and 15–20 percent for women. Restricted diets should not be observed by young, developing people and pregnant or lactating women.

Changing one's diet is very difficult and if it is to succeed one must think of food differently. Start looking at food as a nutritional supplement or as an accompaniment to a ceremonial occasion. Figure out other activities besides meals for socializing. Turn off commercials that continuously encourage you to eat. A whole array of new activities, and lifestyles can emerge.

Let's turn now to a brief review of where the final breakthroughs in regeneration and control of aging will most likely occur.

EUMITOSIS OR CELL PROLIFERATION

Mitosis means cell division. The body is constructed from mitotic cells, which have the natural capability to divide throughout the life span, and postmitotic cells, which do not divide after early development. It is in the postmitotic, nondividing cells that primary aging occurs. A good example of postmitotic cells is the small array of neurons in the midbrain called the *substantia nigra.*

Neurons in the substantia nigra area of the brain appear to be nondividing, postmitotic cells. Several months after birth, they apparently cease having the ability to divide. From that point, no new neurons are created. Neurons do increase in size, however, until their development stops at about age 20. By age 60 or 70, the substantia nigra has aged or deteriorated to a significant extent, and some signs of Parkinson's Disease are usually evident. Several things can be done to slow the aging of the substantia nigra. For example, one can reduce the rate and extent of metabolic wear and tear by following a calorically restricted diet. One can take a proteolytic enzyme inhibitor (Selegiline also known as Deprenyl) to increase availability of the main product of the substantia nigra, dopamine. Deorenyl is a MAO-B inhibitor, which inhibits the enzyme which breaks down dopamine, resulting in higher levels of dopamine. It doesn't increase *production* of dopamine. When the substantia nigra cells cease to function, the dopamine itself can be supplemented. The ultimate cure for the aging of the substantia nigra (and resulting Parkinson's disease), however, and that of all other postmitotic cells would be to induce cells to redivide properly and regenerate their natural population. This process is called eumitosis. For practical purposes, cell division or eumitosis would result in complete regeneration.

During the early 1990s there were almost twenty thousand citations in which "cell proliferation" was the main subject in the Medline data base, which indexes about 70 percent of the world's biomedical research. That is a sizable amount of activity for any subject. If we assume that for each citation there are multiple investigators, then there may be over 40,000 scientists worldwide who are working in this area. Most of the work is focused on cancer because cancer is uncontrolled cell proliferation. Cancer and aging, however, go hand in hand.

More than fifty scientists met in Montreal, Canada, in the early 1990s to compare data and map future directions for research in the area of the "control of cell proliferation in senescent cells." The main topics at that convention were: "Control of DNA Synthesis in Senescent Cells"; "Growth Factors and Signal Transduction"; "Transcriptional Control and RNA Processing"; "Regulatory Pathways and Differentiation"; and "Mapping Senescence Genes."

The meeting was cosponsored by the National Institute on Aging in Bethesda and the Bloomfield Centre for Research in Aging in Montreal. In the funding budget for the National Institute on Aging, cell proliferation research was featured strongly and received substantial funding. Two of the front-line investigators in this field are James R. Smith and Olivia M. Pereira-Smith of Baylor College of Medicine in Houston who have been working in this area for over two decades. Tracking their path will give a good idea of where future research may be headed.

TABLE 10.2 GROWTH FACTOR CITATIONS IN THE MEDLINE DATA BASE

The Growth Factor	Number of Citations
Angiogenesis Factor	125
Cyclins	685
Endothelial Growth Factors	182
Epidermal Growth	3,495
Fibroblast Growth Factor	838
Growth Inhibitors	881
Hematopoietic Cell Growth	872
Hepatocyte Growth Factor	243
Interleukins	936
Maturation-Promoting Factor	161
Nerve Growth Factors	2,189
Neuroleukin	4
Platelet-Derived Growth Factor	1,817
Somatomedins	962
Transforming Growth Factors	515
Biopterin	704
Transforming Growth Factor beta	2,913
Lectins	2,672
Lipopolysaccharides	5,390

Starting with studies on the Hayflick phenomenon of limited cell doubling, Smith and Pereira-Smith were interested in the mechanism of the limitation. In a series of experiments, they fused immortal cell lines that are capable of dividing forever with normal cell lines that have limited division. They found that cellular immortality was inhibited by this fusion. They also discovered that at least two separate events in the normal cell genetic code (genome) can result in the reactivation of immortality. In more recent work, their evidence suggests that DNA synthesis inhibitors are involved in the limited life span of normal cells and that the process of making cells divide indefinitely may involve alterations in the activity of or response to such inhibitors.

The controlled induction of eumitosis will probably be accomplished by the administration of agents called mitogens or "growth factors". To give a flavor for the popularity of this area of science, above is a listing of the main growth factors with the corresponding number of reports filed in Medline in the early 1990s.

The development of growth factors and mitogens as clinically available therapies presents a promising area for research. Cell populations that are deteriorated either from disease or aging may be regenerated. Hopefully, the near future will reveal all of the elusive factors that prevent life shortening disease and maintain biological vitality by means of slowing or reversing biological aging.

CHAPTER ELEVEN

THE LIFE-EXPECTANCY CALCULATION

In this section, you will be making various life-expectancy calculations that apply to you personally. First, you will start with your statistical life expectancy. After that, you will make modifications according to your personal genetics, environment, and behavior. Then you will estimate your revised life expectancy if you implement certain basic life-extension practices. Finally, you will make a series of estimates based on research developments likely to occur over the years to come. These calculations will provide a picture of your current status, the more immediate life-expectancy prospects, and the longer-range life expectancy. If you presently have a serious medical disorder, however, this calculation may not accurately apply to you. Follow the instructions for each of the scenarios that below.

SCENARIO 1: YOUR ACTUARIAL LIFE EXPECTANCY

Because you are from the human species you conform to the general life-span pattern characteristic of that species. In addition, because you live within a particular social and environmental context, your species life span is allowed to express itself according to varying degrees of its full potential. Thus, the first figure to be used in calculating your life span is the actuarial or average life span for humans living within your particular cultural and environmental setting.

What follows are two tables (one for females and the other for males) in which average life expectancies are listed for different age categories. The tables are standard actuarial calculations used by insurance companies, compiled from statistics of the Metropolitan Life Insurance Company in 1979. The figures apply to an average industrialized civilization. We will use this figure as a starting point. Go to your current age in the table and note the number of years of your life expectancy according to your gender.

LIFE EXPECTANCY TABLE 11.1 - FEMALES

Age	Life Span	Age	Life Span	Age	Life Span	Age	Life Span
20	78	35	79	50	80	65	83
21	78	36	79	51	80	66	83
22	78	37	78.9	52	80	67	84
23	78	38	79	53	81	68	84
24	78	39	79	54	81	69	84
25	78	40	79.1	55	80.8	70	84
26	79	41	79.2	56	81	71	85
27	79	42	79.3	57	81	72	85
28	79	43	79.3	58	81	73	85
29	79	44	79.4	59	81.6	74	86
30	79	45	79.5	60	81.8	75	86
31	79	46	79.6	61	82	76	87
32	79	47	79.7	62	82	77	87
33	79	48	79.8	63	83	78	88
34	79	49	80	64	83	79	88

LIFE EXPECTANCY TABLE 11.2 - MALES

Age	Life Span	Age	Life Span	Age	Life Span	Age	Life Span
20	71	35	72.3	50	74.2	65	78.7
21	71.1	36	72.4	51	74.4	66	79.1
22	71.2	37	72.5	52	74.6	67	80
23	71.3	38	72.6	53	74.9	68	80
24	71.4	39	72.7	54	75.1	69	80.5
25	71.5	40	72.8	55	75.4	70	80.9
26	71.6	41	72.9	56	75.6	71	81.4
27	71.7	42	73	57	75.9	72	81.9
28	71.8	43	73.1	58	76.2	73	82.5
29	71.8	44	73.2	59	76.5	74	83
30	71.9	45	73.4	60	76.8	75	83.6
31	72	46	73.5	61	77.2	76	84.2
32	72.1	47	73.7	62	77.5	77	84.8
33	72.2	48	73.9	63	77.9	78	85.4
34	72.2	49	74	64	78.3	79	86.1

Record your actuarial life expectancy here: _____ (1A)
Now, make the following calculation:

$$\underline{\hspace{3cm}} - \underline{\hspace{3cm}} = \underline{\hspace{3cm}}$$

actuarial life   current age   years remaining (1C)
expectancy (1A)   estimate (1B)

The above actuarial life expectancy is a general statistical calculation. To be more precise, personal factors must be accounted for. These will be considered next.

SCENARIO 2: THE EFFECTS OF GENETICS, SOCIAL FACTORS, BEHAVIOR, AND ENVIRONMENT ON YOUR LIFE EXPECTANCY

The following genetic, social, behavioral, and environmental factors are known to relate to your health, your proneness to specific diseases, and your life expectancy. In answering the questions below, make your notations as you read the material. At the end of this section, you will add and subtract the various factors and make an adjustment to your actuarial life expectancy. If you cannot answer a particular question, disregard it.

GENETIC FACTORS

For each grandparent or parent who died of
heart attack or stroke before age 50, subtract
2 years; and for any who died from those diseases
between ages 51 and 60, subtract 1.   -___
If any of your recent ancestors had diabetes,
thyroid disorders, or cancer and you are not
taking special precautions as advised by a
doctor, then subtract 1 year for each disorder.   -___

SOCIAL AND CULTURAL FACTORS

If you live in an average industrialized
society, make no change. If you live in an
advanced technological society,
add 2 years.   +___
If you live in an emerging industrial
society, subtract 5 years.   -___
If you graduated from college, add 1 year.   +___
If you income is over $65,000 per year or
less than $15,000, subtract 2 years.   -___

PERSONAL BEHAVIORAL FACTORS

If most of your life you have maintained
optimal body weight (i.e., you are presently and
have been for some time neither overweight
nor underweight by more than about 5 pounds,
add 5 years. +___

If you are between 12–14 pounds underweight,
subtract 1 year; if 15 or more pounds
underweight, subtract 2 years. -___

If you are overweight, subtract 1 year for
every 10 pounds over your ideal weight. -___

If you skip meals frequently, if you do not
regularly eat two or three meals per day
(including breakfast), and if you eat
hurriedly, then subtract 1 year. -___

Subtract 1 year for each of the following
types of food which you eat routinely:

fast foods -___

refined sugar -___

fatty foods -___

salty foods -___

If you eat at least one meal a day containing
foods from the basic food groups, add 2 years. +___

If you take a multiple vitamin and mineral
daily or extra vitamin A, C, or E, add 1 year. +___

If you eat a high-fiber food daily, add 1
year. +___

If you are a moderate drinker of alcohol
(i.e. 1 glass of wine or 1 cocktail per day),
add 1 year. +___

If you drink alcohol more than 2 drinks per day,
subtract 2 years for every 2 drinks beyond
that. -___

If you frequently sleep fewer than 5 hours
or more than 9 hours, subtract 2 years.   - ___
If you smoke more than 40 cigarettes per day,
subtract 8 years.   - ___
If you smoke 20–40 cigarettes per day   - ___
subtract 6 years.
If you smoke 10–20 cigarettes per day,
subtract 3 years.   - ___
If you do not smoke but live or work with
smokers, subtract 2 years.   - ___
If you exercise for half an hour or more at
least three times per week, add 2 years
(note: only the more strenuous, aerobically
sustained, exercising counts such as swimming,
hiking, racket ball, jogging, etc.).   + ___
If you are sedentary in work and outside of
work, subtract 2 years.   - ___
If you lead a mentally active life, add
1 year.   + ___
If you are often bored and depressed,
subtract 1 year.   - ___
If you are basically happy, add 1 year.   + ___
If you are under chronic emotional stress
and anxiety, subtract 2 years   - ___
If you are calm and easygoing, add 1 year.   + ___
If you are highly aggressive, competitive, or
easily irritated, subtract 1 year   - ___

ENVIRONMENTAL FACTORS

If you live in a polluted environment,
subtract 1 year.   - ___
If you work in a polluted environment,
subtract 3 years.   - ___

PERSONAL BIOMEDICAL FACTORS

If your blood pressure is 130/90, subtract 1 year;
if it is 140/90, subtract 3 years; and if it is
150/100 or greater subtract 5 years.   -___

If you take therapeutic drugs on a prolonged
basis which have known side effects, subtract 2
years.   -___

If your blood cholesterol is 220 or more,
subtract 1 year.   -___

If your HDL cholesterol is low, subtract 1
year.   -___

If you frequently take drugs for recreational
purposes, subtract 2 years.   -___

If you have annual or semi-annual comprehensive
examinations for preventive medicine, add 2 years.   +___

SUMMARIZE THE PREVIOUS FIGURES HERE

The total years added   +___   (2A)
The total years subtracted   -___   (2B)

Next, in order to establish the effects of your genetic, social,
behavioral, and environmental factors on your life expectancy, complete the following calculation.

Your actuarial life expectancy from Scenario 1A ___

plus the total additions from Scenario 2A   +___

minus the subtractions from Scenario 2B   -___

equals your adjusted life expectancy   =___

Scenario 2 represents a fairly reasonable approximation of your personal life expectancy as it stands at this point in time. You are ready now to begin your life extension program in several different phases.

SCENARIO 3: YOUR PHASE I LIFE-EXTENSION PROGRAM

The main objectives of Phase I applications are the optimization of personal behavior, environment, and social factors, and compensation for any particular genetic predisposition to disease. Thus, the first phase of your life-extension program would be to correct as many of the negatives as possible in Scenario 2. You would have routine comprehensive testing at appropriate intervals. Based upon that data you would (a) make certain adjustments in nutrition; (b) begin an exercise program; (c) minimize your exposure to toxins; (d) reduce your anxiety and other psychological factors that cause unnecessary stress; and (e) profile your risk to cancer, heart attack, and other diseases and institute preventive measures.

We will assume that to implement such a program would take you about three years. As a consequence of such changes, you would be able to normalize the negative factors in Scenario 2.

Now, make a modification in your life expectancy by doing the following calculation. From the last adjusted life expectancy in Scenario 2 (page ##), take the total number of years that were subtracted from your life expectancy and add those years to your adjusted life expectancy.

Your adjusted life expectancy from Scenario 2C _____

Add with the total subtractions from Scenario + ___
2C
Equals your Phase I life expectancy: = ___   (3A)

SCENARIO 4: THE BENEFITS FROM EXPECTED PROGRESS IN BASIC RESEARCH

From this point, we will be making conjectures about progress that is likely to occur in life-extension and control of aging research.

SCENARIO 4A: WITHIN THE NEXT 5 YEARS

Let's assume that within the next five years you will be able to establish a routine diet that is calorically restricted. Your average daily intake will be about 1,800 calories. In addition, some progress will have occurred in the life-extension sciences. For example, technology in curative medicine and disease prevention by the early detection of disorders and early therapeutic intervention will have improved considerably. Phase I applications in nutrition, exercise, toxicology, and stress management will also have become more refined and more integrated into your lifestyle. The net result of these relatively modest accomplishments in health management will increase and help maintain your vitality such that an additional eighteen years would be added to your life expectancy.

Modify your life expectancy by the following calculation:
Your Phase I Life Expectancy from Scenario 3A ____

plus 18 years from Scenario 4A   +18
equals your revised Life Expectancy: = ____   (4A)

SCENARIO 4B: WITHIN THE NEXT 10 YEARS

Assume that, in ten years from the present, progress continues. The previous procedures become more refined. Also, individual hormonal monitoring and supplementation will be routine; cardiovascular disease will be more preventable and repairable; cancer treatment and prevention techniques, more developed; and individualized nutrition will have developed into a true science. Further, some of the life-extension and gerontological research which began in the 1950s and 1960s will start to surface in the form of applied therapies. For example, a truly effective antioxidant compound will have been certified and be available for use, and there will be effective pharmacological management of some aspects of mental aging. As a result of that progress, your vitality will be improved such that another fifteen years will be added to your life expectancy.

Modify your life expectancy accordingly:
Your Scenario 4A life expectancy   _____

Plus 15 years from Scenario 4B   + 15
Equals your revised Life Expectancy: = ___   (4B)

SCENARIO 4C: WITHIN THE NEXT 20 YEARS

As time progresses, the involvement in and support of aging research will have grown, and the systematic mapping of the basic mechanisms of regeneration will have yielded major progress. The stage is set for major breakthroughs. Assume that, during the next twenty years, new developments continue. All of the previous techniques continue to become more refined and more effective, yielding additional maintenance of vitality. Also, there will be available rudimentary methods for regeneration, such as: methods to stimulate the synthesis of certain types of proteins which degrade with time. Perhaps, as some investigators believe, it is found that the aging of certain systems is caused by inhibiting hormones; and agents are developed which block those inhibiting hormones. Also, it may be discovered that there are, in fact, defects in receptor sites to thyroid hormone and that those defects can be corrected, thus returning general metabolism back to a more optimal state. Those are, of course, speculative; but it is highly probable that within the next twenty years, the aging processes will be under some control. Such progress will yield additional increments in vitality and extensions in life expectancy, giving another twenty years.

Modify your calculation accordingly:
Your Scenario 4B life expectancy   ____

Plus 20 years from Scenario 4C   + 20
Equals your revised Life Expectancy: = ____   (4D)

SCENARIO 4D: WITHIN THE NEXT 30 YEARS

In thirty years from now, the life-extension and control-of-aging sciences will have developed even further, and we should be on the way to achieving the final breakthroughs. In addition to continued refinements of those areas which have been mentioned previously, we will be able to do more basic biological regeneration. Such techniques as monoclonal antibody production and clonal restoration of stem cells will allow us to augment and/or restore the immune system, thus avoiding a host of associated diseases and biological damage. There will be agents to stabilize the repair of the master genetic molecule, DNA, and to regenerate mitochondria. Such breakthroughs will significantly stabilize and regenerate vitality and add about thirty additional years to one's life expectancy.

Modify your calculation accordingly:
Your Scenario 4C life expectancy   ____

plus 30 years from Scenario 4D   + 30
equals your revised Life Expectancy: = ____   (4D)

SCENARIO 4E: WITHIN THE NEXT 40 YEARS

Finally, within forty years, there should be agents that enable the controlled reactivation of cell division in the nonrenewable or post-mitotic types of cells. Once that type of technology is accomplished, complete biological regeneration will, most likely, be possible; and we will have the ability to reverse and control aging and maintain optimal vitality indefinitely through time. For all practical purposes, that will be tantamount to scientific "immortality"; and that is the inevitable goal of medicine and the ultimate goal of the life-extension sciences. Once this level of technology is reached, then you would be a nonaging human, functioning in a physical condition of optimal vitality, and your potential would be open-ended. From that point on, only periodic regeneration would be required to biologically maintain you at that level of optimal vitality; and your life expectancy would be potentially indefinite.

Keep in mind that the last scenarios are speculative and depend on progress in the biological sciences. It could be argued that those predictions are overly optimistic; but it could be argued, with equal validity, that they are too conservative. The history of modern science demonstrates very clearly that virtually any problem can be solved and any barrier overcome and that breakthroughs frequently happen much sooner that most people think, including the experts. The rate limiting factor on our progress is mostly the amount and manner of applied resources. While the amount of available resources is always a problem, equally significant are the barriers which are self-imposed by the limits of our aspiration and imagination.

The Life-Expectancy Calculation © Foundation for Infinite Survival, Inc., Life Extension & Control of Aging Program, P.O. Box 5875-C, Berkeley, California 94705. Internet address: http://www.fis.org

CHAPTER TWELVE

LIFE EXTENSION—THE WAVE OF THE FUTURE

This book reviews the current state of knowledge in the field of life extension and control of aging. Information is provided so the reader is supplied with the knowledge necessary to differentiate between ineffective and effective solutions. The importance of proof for any claims for longevity-resulting products is discussed in this final chapter.

Life-extension science has evolved out of the realm of myth and folk medicine to emerge as a rigorous science. The progress in life-extension science is linked to general progress in many areas of molecular biology. Who knows what surprises the future may bring! Important areas to watch include breakthroughs in the finalization of genetic mapping and proof of cytoplasmic involvement in the control of cell regeneration.

When mapping of human genetic material is complete, we should then have a good idea about which particular genes are instrumental in the construction and operation of all cellular functions. At that point, focus can be directed to specific genes to induce desired effect. The mechanism of cell regeneration is also key to the future of life-extension science. Richard Strohman of the University of California at Berkeley has for years maintained the primacy of cytoplasmic mechanisms. Judging from current work in cell proliferation, it appears that mitosis is indeed regulated in the cytoplasm of the cell.

MORE AND MORE PEOPLE LIVING LONGER

In the mid-1990s in the United States alone, there were over 33 million people over age 65, with over 20% of this population needing help with such essentials as bathing and getting out of bed. As the percentage of aging individuals continues to increase, the demand for solutions will intensify. There will be more and more advertising for products and services attempting to meet this demand. These products and services will claim to be beneficial for life extension and control of aging. Hopefully the information provided in this book will equip you to differentiate between substantive approaches, which can have some tangible benefit, and approaches that are likely to be ineffective. Here is a set of simple guidelines to help evaluate claims.

GUIDELINES FOR EVALUATING
LIFE-EXTENSION CLAIMS

First, an assertion or claim made or implied in a scientific study, experiment, or journal does not necessarily mean much. Scientific journals do have a "peer review" process in an attempt to avoid publishing information that is obviously incorrect or misconstrued. However, the nature of good science is to be fairly open and allow for a wide range of varying and conflicting ideas. The process of replication and discourse is supposed to weed out what is erroneous. This dialectical process takes time. To follow and understand it requires a fairly well-developed acumen in the specialized semantics of a particular discipline. Thus, when you see that such and such a scientist has found that agent "X" extends the life span or slows aging, that is just an entrée for you to begin asking critical questions.

Learn to say, "May I see the data please?" A life extensionist must not be intimidated by the authoritarian mantle that the term "scientist" commonly evokes.

If a claim is one of "life extension," it is important to ask and obtain answers to a number of questions. The answers to the following questions are important to help judge the effectiveness of any experiments performed. All of the following inquiries are included in the questionnaire provided in Appendix C. Appendix C also includes a cover letter. You may copy and send the sample letter and questionnaire to the scientists or the company selling any purported life-extension products, or use it as a model to develop your own letter and questionnaire.

MAY I SEE THE DATA, PLEASE?

- What is the technical name of the experimental agent?
- If a chemical, what is the Chemical Abstracts Service registry number?(CAS#)?
- In what animal model was the experiment done?
- Is this a genetically well-characterized model that most gerontologists would agree is suitable for life-span studies?
- What percent of control animals survived? How many days?
- What percent of the experimentals survived? How many days?
- Were the body weights of the experimental animals comparable to the controls at the beginning?
- Were the body weights of the experimental animals comparable to the controls at the end?
- Is it likely that the life extension was the result of caloric restriction?
- Are the survival data or rates of your controls the same as or better than the survival data and rates of other investigators with this strain?

Any worthwhile researcher in life-extension science will have all of these details and be able to relay them rapidly. Once you receive the survival data from the questionnaire, plot the data on a survival curve. Does the data reflect Phase I life extension or Phase II life extension?

If the body weights of the experimental animals were lower than the body weights of the controls, it is possible the agent being tested caused the food to taste bad. As a result the experimental animals will have eaten less. That means they were calorically restricted, the probable cause of the life extension. This is a common fallacy in life-extension experiments.

If the researcher's controls lived suboptimally, it is possible that the agent being tested compensated for some life-shortening aspect of the environment and the life extension in the experimentals was apparent but not real. This is another common artifact in these studies.

If the experiment was done in humans, then the questionnaire does not apply. The life-extension claim will probably be based on the improvement of some biomarker of aging or health. A common dilemma arises from these studies. Often the experimental and control groups have a deficiency (as was the case in the testosterone experiment quoted in Chapter 6). If the agent being tested made an improvement in some biological or psychological marker, the most likely interpretation is that the agent compensated for a deficiency. Claims of benefit would only apply to those who have that particular deficiency, and probably would not help humans who have sufficient amounts of the substance being tested.

Serious life extensionists do not have the time, money, or energy to spend on ineffective or palliative measures. It is better to do nothing than to do something superfluous or detrimental. There is plenty to do in the next few years to create a general lifestyle following the practices already described in this book. Following these simple practices may help you to position yourself ecologically and socially for the monumental transitions that have already begun.

To live as long as Methuselah supposedly lived may never be in the realm of possibility. Living to the age of 120 is possible at this point in time, however, and steps which could help you achieve this goal in a vibrant and energetic state have been presented in this book. Hopefully the secrets of life extension will be revealed sometime in the next century, and those of us who wish to will be around to reap the benefits of what the future has in store. In the meantime, take care of your health, and approach new methods of life extension with extreme caution.

APPENDIX A

ROY WALFORD'S CALORIC-RESTRICTION STUDIES

To encapsulate the portion of Walford's work that relates to caloric restriction, the following summary of citations is provided. These are only his work vis a vis caloric restriction; his research in other areas of immunology and aging is impressive, but due to space limitations is not included. These citations are ordered chronologically.

In the footnoting of scientific research papers mentioned, a modern technique of bibliographic referencing citation, called a "unique identification number" (UIN) is provided. The UIN identifies each specific report in the Medline data base. Anyone interested in greater detail can use these numbers to retrieve an abstract of the report cited. Unfortunately, the unique identification numbers are not available for research prior to 1966. Books also do not have unique identification numbers.

A Partial List of Roy Walford's Work Regarding Caloric Restriction

Name of Research Paper	UIN
Long-term dietary restriction and immune function in mice: response to sheep red blood cells and to mitogenic agents.	74252427
Immune function and survival in a long-lived mouse strain subjected to undernutrition.	76044556
Influence of controlled dietary restriction on immunologic function and aging.	79169935
Survival and disease patterns in C57BL/6J mice subjected to undernutrition.	81004188
Modification of mitochondrial respiration by aging and dietary restriction.	80231268
Immunology and aging [Philip Levine Award].	81018974
Influence of weaning-initiated dietary restriction on responses to T cell mitogens and on splenic T cell levels in a long-lived F1-hybrid mouse strain.	82236016
Modification of age-related immune decline in mice dietarily restricted from or after midadulthood.	82151003
Dietary restriction in mice beginning at 1 year of age: effect on lifespan and spontaneous cancer incidence.	82152762
Influence of dietary restriction and aging on natural killer cell activity in mice.	83084017
The effect of dietary restriction of varying duration on survival, tumor patterns, immune function, and body temperature in B10C3F1 female mice.	83239632

Continued on next page…

Name of Research Paper	UIN
Food intake reduction and immunologic alterations in mice fed dehydro-epiandrosterone.	85076847
Dietary restriction retards age-related loss of gamma crystallins in the mouse lens.	84223927
The extension of maximum life span.	86161253
The retardation of aging in mice by dietary restriction: longevity, cancer, immunity and lifetime energy intake.	86170833
Dietary restriction benefits learning and motor performance of aged mice.	87084516
Influences of dietary restriction and age on liver enzyme activities and lipid peroxidation in mice.	87168767
Dietary restriction and aging: historical phases, mechanisms and current directions.	88035259
The 120-year diet [letter].	88103386
Influences of aging and dietary restriction on serum thymosin alpha 1 levels in mice.	88154337
The retardation of aging and disease by dietary restriction.	A book No UIN
Caloric restriction perturbs the pituitary-ovarian axis and inhibits mouse mammary tumor virus production in a high-spontaneous-mammary-tumor-incidence mouse strain (C3H/SHN).	90013440
How dietary restriction retards aging: an integrative hypothesis [editorial].	90292775
The clinical promise of diet restriction.	90201707
Dietary restriction alone and in combination with oral ethoyquin/2-mercaptoethylamine in mice.	90369121
Dietary energy restriction in mice reduces hepatic expression of glucose-regulated protein 78 (BiP) and 94 mRNA.	91038376
Lack of effect of age and dietary restriction on DNA single-stranded breaks in brain, liver, and kidney of (C3H x C57BL/10) F1 mice.	91147688
Influence of age and caloric restriction on expression of hepatic genes for xenobiotic and oxygen metabolizing enzymes in the mouse.	91231682
Influences of dietary restriction on immunity to influenza in aged mice.	91302705
Influence of age and caloric restriction on macrophage IL-6 and TNF production.	92118990
Aging and restriction of dietary calories increases insulin receptor mRNA, & aging increases glucocorticoid receptor mRNA in the liver of female C3B10RF1 mice.	92043328
Dietary restriction maintains linoleic and arachidonic acid levels in murine liver during aging.	93042068
Specific inhibition of pituitary prolactin production by energy restriction in C3H/SHN female mice.	92333957
Failure of dietary restriction to retard age-related neurochemical changes in mice.	93149339
The calorically restricted low-fat nutrient-dense diet in Biosphere 2 significantly lowers blood glucose, total leukocyte count, cholesterol, and blood pressure in humans.	93087562
Effect of age and extent of dietary restriction on hepatic microsomal lipid peroxidation potential in mice.	94202985

APPENDIX B: AGING MEASUREMENT SERVICES				
TEST NAME	NOTES	COMPANY AVAILABLE FROM	COMPANY ADDRESS	COMPANY PHONE NUMBER
DIAGNOSTIC & EVALUATORY TESTS	Hair analysis for tissue minerals, EMA™, computerized diet analysis	The American College of Advancement in Medicine	PO Box 3427 Laguna Hills, CA 92654	714-583-7666
ADRENAL STRESS INDEX	Test kits & instructions for conducting the test.	Diagnos-Techs Incorporated	6620 S 192nd Pl Suite J-104 Kent, WA 98032	800-878-3787
BASAL METABOLIC RATE AND SERUM LIPID PEROXIDE LEVELS	The whole-body calorimeter that measures the test	Basal-Tech Incorporated	726 Lafayette Ave Cincinnati, OH 45220	513-751-2723
INDIVIDUAL DIET ANALYSIS	Information on individualized diet analysis	Dr. Walford's Interactive Diet Planner LongBrook Co.	1015 Gayley Ave #1215 Los Angeles, CA 90024	
COMPUTER DIET ANALYSIS	Information on computerized diet analysis	Life Extension & Control of Aging Program	PO Box 4000-C Berkeley, CA 94704	
CROSS-LINKING INDEX	Serum assay that measures the degree of intermolecular cross-linking	Metra Biosystems Incorporated	3181 Porter Dr Palo Alto, CA 94304	415-494-9114
ESSENTIAL METABOLICS	Blood samples are collected in two 10-milliliter heparinized tubes	Spectracell Labs Incorporated	515 Post Oak Blvd Suite 830 Houston, TX 77027	713-621-3101 800-227-5227
HANDYGRIP DYNAMOMETER		Lafayette Instrument Co	PO Box 5729 Lafayette, IN 47903	
HAIR ANALYSIS	Samples must be submitted through your physician	Life Extension & Control of Aging Program	PO Box 4000 Berkeley, CA 94704	
INFORMATION ON OTHER TESTS	Scientists are developing tests to figure out composite biological ages	Ward Dean, M.D. The Center for Bio-Gerontology	PO Box 11097 Pensacola, FL 32524	

APPENDIX C
EXPERIMENTAL QUESTIONNAIRE FOR LIFE-EXTENSION

The technical name of the experimental agent is

If a chemical, the CAS# is _____

In what animal model was the experiment done? _____

Is this a genetically, well-characterized model that most gerontologists would agree is suitable for life-span studies?

Please provide the following survival data:

100%		100%	
90%		90%	
80%		80%	
70%		70%	
60%		60%	
50%		50%	
40%		40%	
30%		30%	
20%		20%	
10%		10%	
0%		0%	

Were the body weights of the experimental animals comparable to the controls? _____

At the beginning? _____

At the end? _____

Is it likely that the life extension was the result of caloric restriction? _____

Are the survival data or rates of your controls the same as or better than the survival data and rates of other investigators with this strain? _____

LETTER TO SCIENTISTS

Feel free to copy and send the following model letter and question-naire on the previous page to the scientists or the company selling products purporting life extension, or use it as a model to develop your own letter and questionnaire.

From: _____   Date: _____

_____

_____

_____

To: _____

_____

_____

_____

Regarding the claim of life extension for _____

_____

I am very interested in this work and would greatly appreciate answers to the following questions. If you have a report that already addresses these issues, please send a reprint.

Thank you,

_____

APPENDIX D
SUPPLIERS AND SERVICES

These listings are provided for information purposes only and are not recommendations by the authors or the publisher. Most suppliers and services will respond to inquiries about specific products only. Some suppliers offer price lists and order forms upon request. To obtain more information or to order, write or call for ordering information, availability, current prices, and shipping charges. The authors and publisher recommend that readers consult with their physicians before using any products supplied by these companies or any other suppliers.

• Alzheimer's Buyers Club, Box 7006, San Jose 1000, Costa Rica. Organized by Dr. William Summers. Supplies THA and lecithin.

• American College of Advancement in Medicine, Box 3427, Laguna Hills, CA 92654. 714-583-7666 or 800-532-3688. Maintains a list of physicans with expertise in life extension and cognative enhancement.

• B. Mougios & Co. O.E., Pittakou 23 T. K., 54645, Thessaloniki, Greece. Supplies most nootropics.

• Baxamed Switzerland Medical Center, Realpstrasse 83, CH-4054 Basel, Switzerland, FAX 061-301-38-72. Supplies smart pharmaceuticals by mail order.

• Big Ben Export Co., Tudor Trading Co., P.O. Box 146, Mill Hill, London NW7 3DL, England. Supplies many smart pharmeceuticals that can be ordered with Visa and Mastercard.

• Cell Tech, 1300 Main St., Klamath Falls, OR. 97601, 503-882-5406. Suppliers of Super Blue-Green™ microalgae products.

• Center for Bio-Gereontology, publishes Biological Aging Measurement: Clinical Applications by Ward Dean M.D., P.O. Box 11097, Pensacola, FL 32524.

• J. Channet, MD, Postfach, CH-891, Rifferswil, Switzerland. Supplies KH-3.

• Discovery Experimental & Development, Mexico, N.A., B & B Freight Forwarding Service, Inc., P.O. Box 7178, Wesley Chapel, FL 33543; Mexico: 011-5266-304464. Supplies liquid deprenyl which can be ordered COD by phone for 5–7 day UPS delivery.

• Foundation for Infinite Survival, P.O. Box 5875, Berkeley, CA 94705; World Wide Web Address: http://www.fis.org

• Gerovital, Inc., Beverly Hills, CA; 800-833-9834. Residential program providing traditional Ana Aslan treatment.

• GH-7 Product Literature, 1920 Monument Blvd. #544, Concord, CA 95420.

• J-M Pharmacal Co. 251-B East Hacienda Ave., Campbell, CA 95008, 408-374-5920, 800-538-4545. Wholesalers of amino acids. Customers can phone for a product and price list.

• Life Extension Foundation, 995 SW 24th St., Ft. Lauderdale, FL 33315; Box 229120, Hollywood, FL 33022; 305-966-4886, 800-841-5433. Members receive monthly newsletter; Helpful directories to life extension doctors and innovative medical clinics. Membership is $50.

• Life Services Supplements, Inc., 81 First Avenue, Atlantic Highlands, NJ 07716; 800-542-3230; 908-872-8700; Fax 908-872-8705. Sells Pearson and Shaw products and offers distributorships.

• Longevity Plus Buyer's Club, U Dubu 27, 147 00 Prague 4-Branik, Czechoslovakia. Supplies many smart pharmaceuticals and accepts personal checks. Will send an order form upon request.

• Masters Marketing Co. Ltd., Masters House, No. 1 Marlborough Hill, Harrow Middx., HA1 1TW, England, Fax 081-427-1994. Supplies a wide range of smart pharmaceuticals and other products. Interested persons must write or Fax specifying information on specific products for a price quotation.

• Mexican pharmacies supply nootropics over the counter without a prescription and are usually less expensive than ordering by mail order.

• Nutrient Café Smart Drinks, Chris Beaumont, Box 170156, San Francisco, CA 94117. 415-267-6178. Provides a smart bar with smart drinks for events. Offers a smart bar recipe book for $2.

• Qwilleran, Box 1210, Birmingham, B10 9QA, England. Supplies most nootropics and some AIDS drugs. Inquiries must specify the products you are interested in.

• Smart Products, 1626 Union Street, San Francisco, CA 94123; Phone: 1 800-878-6520; Fax 415.351.1348 Supplies smart nutrient products. Orders can be placed by phone with credit card or by mail with personal check or drop in. Discounts on orders over $100 and two day delivery is available. Monthly newsletter. Sells DHEA. World Wide Web Address: http://www.smartbasic.com

• Dr. William Summers, 624 West Duarte Rd., Suite 101, Arcadia, CA 91007; 818-445-6196; Fax 818-445-4204. Works with families of Alzheimer's patients and affiliated with the Alzheimer's Buyers Club.

• Sun Wellness Inc., 4025 Spencer St #104, Torrance CA 90503; 1.800.829.2828. or 310.371.5515. Suppliers of chlorella microalgae products.

• Wholesale Nutrition, Box 3345, Saratoga, CA 95070, 800-325-2664; FAX 408-867-6236. Supplies smart nutrients. Orders can be placed by phone with credit card. Two day delivery is available.

• World Health Services, P.O. Box 20, CH-2822 Courroux, Switzerland. Supplies many European pharmaceuticals that have not been approved by the FDA.

APPENDIX E

ORGANIZATIONS AND INFORMATION CENTERS

•*Aging and Degenerative Disease Research,* Pharmaceutical Products Division, Abbott Laboratories Abbott Park, IL 60064.

•Aging and Dementia Research Center New York University Medical Center, Millhauser Laboratories, New York, NY 10016.

•*Aging Studies Branch Centers for Disease Control and Prevention* Atlanta, GA

•Aging Study Unit of the Geriatric Research, Education and Clinical Center Veterans Affairs Medical Center Palo Alto, Calif 94304.

•Aging Research and Education Center, University of Texas Health Science Center, San Antonio, Texas 78284.

•*Arizona Research Laboratories,* Division of Neural Systems, Memory and Aging, University of Arizona, Tucson, Arizona 85724.

•Aging Study Unit VA Medical Center Palo Alto, CA 94307.

•Allegheny County Department of Aging, Pittsburgh, PA.

•*American Federation for Aging Research,* New York, NY.

•*Bloomfield Centre for Research in Aging,* Lady Davis Institute for Medical Research, Sir Mortimer B. Davis-Jewish General Hospital, Montreal, Quebec, Canada.

•Borun Center for Gerontological Research, UCLA School of Medicine Jewish Home for the Aging Reseda, CA

•*Buck Center for Research on Aging* 505 A San Marin Dr. Novato, CA 94945.

•Center on Aging University of Texas Medical Branch Galveston, TX 77555.

•Center for Aging University of Medicine and Dentistry of New Jersey-School of Osteopathic Medicine Stratford, New Jersey 08084.

•Centre for Studies of Aging University of Toronto; Toronto, Ontario, Canada.

•Center for Research and Study of Aging School of Social Work,, Haifa University, Israel.

•Center for the Study of Aging and Human Development Duke University Durham, NC.

•*Claude D. Pepper Center for Research on Oral Health* University of Florida Health Sciences Center, Gainesville, FL 32610-0416.

•Department of Pharmacology and Therapeutics McGill Center for Studies in Aging Montreal, Quebec, Canada.

•Department of Aging and Mental Health, Florida Mental Health Institute, University of South   Florida Tampa, FL 33612.

•Department of Demyelinating Disease and Aging, National Institute of Neuroscience, Tokyo, Japan. Division on Aging Harvard Medical School, Boston, MA.

•*Foundation for Infinite Survival, Inc.* Life-Extension & Control of Aging Program P.O. Box 5875 Berkeley, CA.

•Free Radical Biology and Aging Research Program Oklahoma Medical Research Foundation Oklahoma City, OK 73104.

•Genetics and Aging Unit, Massachusetts General Hospital-East, Harvard Medical School, Charlestown 02129.

•Gerontology Research Center, National Institute on Aging, Baltimore, Maryland, 21224.

•Gerontology Research Department, Italian National Research Centres on Aging, Ancona, Italy.

•*Global Action on Aging,* New York, NY 10025.

•Huffington Center on Aging, Baylor College of Medicine, Houston, Texas 77030.

•Institute for Biomedical Aging Research of the Austrian Academy of Sciences, Innsbruck, Austria.

•Institute for Brain Aging and Dementia, University of California, Irvine, CA 92717.

•Institute for Health and Aging, University of California, San Francisco CA

•Institute for Health, Health Care Policy and Aging Research, Rutgers University, New Brunswick, NJ 08903.

•Institute of Development, Aging, and Cancer Tohoku University Sendai, Japan.

•Institute on Aging University of Wisconsin-Madison, Madison, WI 53706.

•International Foundation for Biomedical Aging Research, Temple, TX 76503.

•Irvine Research Unit in Brain Aging, University of California, Irvine, CA.

•Japan Institute for Control of Aging, Shizuoka, Japan.

•Jean Mayer US Dept. of Agriculture Human Nutrition Research Center on Aging Tufts Unversity Boston, MA,.

•Laboratory of Molecular Regulation of Aging, Institute of Physical and Chemical Research (RIKEN) Ibaraki, Japan.

•Multidisciplinary Center for the Study of Aging Old Westbury Neuroscience Research Institute, State University of New York New York, NY 11568.

•Menorah Park Center for Aging, Cleveland, Ohio, USA

•Multidisciplinary Center for the Study of Aging Old Westbury Neuroscience Research Institute State University of New York at Old Westbury New York 11568.

•National Institute on Aging, National Institutes of Health, Bethesda, MD 20892.

•*Oasi Institute for Research on Mental Retardation and Brain Aging* Troina, Italy.

•Program on Aging *La Jolla Cancer Research Foundation,* La Jolla, CA 92037.

•Program on Aging, School of Medicine, University of North Carolina Chapel Hill, NC 27599.

•Program on Aging and Applied Gerontology Chicago Medical School, Chicago, IL.

•Research Program in Aging, Sunnybrook Health Science Centre, University of Toronto, North York, Ontario, Canada.

•Research Centre for Aging and Adaptation, Shinshu University School of Medicine Matsumoto, Japan.

•Research Center for Aging and Adaptation Shinshu University School of Medicine Nagana, Japan.

•Research Triangle Institute Program on Aging and Long-Term Care Research Triangle Park, NC 27709.

•*Robarts Research Institute* Department of Stroke and Aging London, Ontario Canada.

•Rehabilitation Engineering Research Center on Aging State University of New York at Buffalo.

•*Rush Institute on Aging* Chicago, IL 60612.

•Sam and Rose Stein Institute for Research on Aging   University of California at San Diego La Jolla, CA 92093-0663.

•Sanders-Brown Research Center on Aging, University of Kentucky, Lexington, Kentucky 40536-0230.

•Stroke Program of the Sanders-Brown Center of Excellence in Aging, University of Kentucky College of Medicine, Lexington, Kentucky 40536.

•*TNO-Institute for Aging and Vascular Research* Leiden, The Netherlands.

•University of Colorado, Center on Aging, Denver, CO 80262.

•University of Texas Medical Branch Center on Aging Galveston, TX.

SUGGESTED READING

NEWSLETTERS

• *Brain/Mind Bulletin*, 4047 San Rafael, Los Angeles, CA, 90065; 213-342-9937.

• *Center For Science in the Public Interest.*1875 Connecticut Ave., N.W. Washington, D.C. 20009.

• *Consumer Reports on Health* P.O. Box 52148 Boulder, CO 80321.

• *Forefront Health Investigations: The Journal of Theoretical and Applied Health Technologies*, Steven Wm. Fowkes, Editor, MegaHealth Society, Box 60637, Palo Alto, CA, 94306; 415-949-0919.

• *Harvard Health Letter* P.O Box 420300 Palm Coast, FL 32142.

• *Intelli-Scope: The Newsletter of the Designer Foods Network*, Smart Products, 870 Market Street, Suite 1262, San Francisco, CA, 94102; 415-981-3334.

• *Life Extension Report*, Saul Kent, Publisher, Box 229120, Hollywood, FL, 33022; 305-966-4886.

• *Life Enhancement News* Will Block, Publisher, P.O. Box 75130, Petaluma, CA 94975. 800-543.3873; Fax 707-769-8016.

• *Mayo Clinic Health Letter* P.O. Box 53889 Boulder, CO 80322.

• *Nootropic News*, John Leslie, Editor, P.O. Box 177, Camarillo, CA, 93011.

• *Smart Drug News: The Newsletter of the Cognitive Enhancement Research Institute*, CERI, Box 4029-4002, Menlo Park, CA, 94026; 415-321-2374; Fax 415-323-3864.

• *Tufts University Diet and Nutrition Letter* P.O Box 57857 Boulder, CO 80322.--

• *University of California Berkeley Wellness Letter* P.O Box 420148 Palm Coast, FL 32142.

BOOKS

• Andersen, K.L., et al., *Fundamentals of Exercise Testing*, World Health Organization, 1978.

• Bjorksten, J., "Cross Linkage and the Aging Process," *Theoretical Aspects of Aging* (Rothstein, M., ed.), pp. 43, 1974.

• Bland, J., "Antioxidants in Nutritional Medicine: Tocopherol, Selenium and Glutathione," *1984–85 Yearbook of Nutritional Medicine*, pp. 213–236, 1985.

• Boyd, R., "Average Weights of Human Body and Brain: Philosophical Transactions of the Royal Society," *Handbook of the Biology of Aging* (1st ed., Finch, C.E. and Hayflick, L., eds.), pp. 242, Van Nostrand Reinhold, 1977.

• Calbom, C. and Keane, M., *Juicing for Life*, Avery Publishing Group, 1992.

• Carper, J., *Stop Aging Now! The Ultimate Plan for Staying Young and Reversing the Aging Process*, HarperCollins, 1995.

• Dean, W., *Biological Aging Measurement: Clinical Applications*, Center for Bio-Gerontology, 1992.

• Dean, W. and Morganthaler, J., *Smart Drugs and Nutrients*, Smart Publications, 1991.

• Dilman, V.M. and Dean, W., *Neuroendocrine Theory of Aging and Degenerative Disease*, Center for Bio-Gerontology, 1992.

• Dimond, M., *Enriching Heredity: The Impact of the Environment on the Anatomy of the Brain*, Center for Bio-Gerontology, 1992.

• *Directory of Life Extension Nutrients and Drugs*, Life Extension International, 1992.

• *Directory of Life Extension Doctors*, Life Extension Foundation, 1992.

• Erdmann, R., *The Amino Revolution*, Simon and Schuster, 1987.

•Dow, Alastair *Deprenyl: The Anti-Aging Drug,* Hallberg Publishing Corp. Clearwater, FL, 1993.

•Everone, C.A., *Life-Extension and Control of Aging Program: Manual of Principles and Procedures,* Foundation for Infinite Survival, 1981.

•Finch, C.E. and Landfield, P.W., "Neuroendocrine and Autonomic Functions in Aging Mammals," *Handbook of the Biology of Aging* (2nd ed., Finch, C.E. and Schneider, E.L., eds.), pp. 567, Van Nostrand Reinhold, 1985.

•Gascoigne, B. and Irwin, J., *Smart Ways to Stay Young and Healthy,* Ronin Publishing, 1992.

•Gillibrand, D., Grewal, D., and Blatter, "Chemistry Reference Values as a Function of Age and Sex, Including Pediatric and Geriatric Subjects," *Aging: Its Chemistry* (Dietz, A.A., ed.), American Association for Clinical Chemistry, pp. 366-389, 1979.

•Gompertz, B., "On the Nature of the Function Expressive of the Law of Human Mortality and on a New Mode of Determining Life Contingencies," *Philosophical Transactions of the Royal Society,* pp. 513-585, 1825.

•Guyton, A.C., *Textbook of Medical Physiology* (7th ed.), W.B. Saunders Company, 1986.

•Haire, N., *Rejuvenation,* Allen and Unwin, 1924.

•Hitchcox, L., *Long Life Now: Strategies for Staying Alive,* Celestial Arts, 1996.

•Hoffer, A. and Walker, M., *Smart Nutrients: A Guide to Nutrients that Can Enhance Intelligence and Reverse Senility,* Avery Publishing, 1993.

•Kaufman, Richard C, Rawson Assoc, New York, 1986

•Kesssler, D., *Caring for the Elderly: Reshaping Health Policy,* John Hopkins Univ. Press

•Keeton, K, *Longevity: The Science of Staying Young,* Viking Penguin, 1992.

•Lehninger, A.L., *Biochemistry* (2nd ed.), pp. 503, Worth Publishers, 1979.

•Mann, J., *Secrets of Life Extension: How to Halt or Reverse the Aging Process and Live a Long and Healthy Life,* And/Or Press and Harbor Publishing, 1980.

•Mark, V. and Mark, J., *Reversing Memory Loss: Proven methods for Regaining, Strengthening, and Preserving Memory,* Houghton Mifflin Company, 1992.

•Montgomery, Rex, et al., *Biochemistry: A Case-Oriented Approach* (3rd ed.), C. V. Mosby Co., pp. 218, 1980.

•Morgan, R. F. and WIlson, J., *Growing Younger,* Methunen, 1983.

•Null, G. and Feldman, M., *Reverse the Aging Process Naturally,* Villard Books, 1993.

•Pearson, D. and Shaw, S., *Life Extension: A Practical Scientific Approach,* Warner Books, 1982.

•Pelton, R., *Mind Foods and Smart Pills,* Doubleday, 1989.

•Pierpaoli, Walter, M.D., Ph D. and Regelson, William M.D. *The Melatonin Miracle,* Simon & Schuster 1995.

•Potter, B. and Orfali, S., *Brain Boosters: Foods and Drugs That Make You Smarter,* Ronin Publishing, 1993.

•Rockstein, Morris, et al, "Comparative Biology and Evolution of Aging," *Handbook of the Biology of Aging* (1st ed., Finch, C.E. and Hayflick, L., eds.), pp. 9, Van Nostrand Reinhold, 1977.

•Rosenfeld, A., *Prolongevity II: An Updated Report on the Scientific Aspects of Adding Good Years to Life,* Henry Holt, 1985.

•Sekuler, R., "Vision as a Source of Simple and Reliable Markers for Aging," *Biomarkers of Aging* (Reff, M. E. and Schneider, E. L., eds.), pp. 226.

•Shock, N.W., "Systems Integration," *Handbook of the Biology of Aging* (1st ed., Finch, C.E. and Hayflick, L., eds.), pp. 639, Van Nostrand Reinhold, 1977.

•Strain, W.H., *Age*, Journal of the American Aging Association, 1978.

•Tortora, G.J. and Anagnostakos, N.P., *Principles of Anatomy and Physiology* (4th ed.), Harper and Row Publishers, 1984.

•Tortora, G.J., Funke, B.R. and Case, C.L., *Microbiology: an Introduction* (2nd ed.), Benjamin/Cummings Publishing, 1986.

•Walford, R.L., *Immunologic Theory of Aging*, Munksgaard, 1969.

•Walford, R.L., *The 120-Year Diet: How to Double Your Vital Years*, Simon and Shuster, 1988.

•Walford, R.L. and Walford, L., *The Anti-Aging Plan: Strategies and Recipes for Extending Your Healthy Years*, Four Walls Eight Windows, 1994.

•Weil, A., *Natural Health, Natural Medicine: A Comprhensive Manual for Wellness and Self-Care*, Houghton Mifflin Company, 1990.

•Weindruch, R. and Walford, R.L., *Retardation of Aging and Disease by Dietary Restriction*, Charles C. Thomas, 1988.

•Wolfe, S.L., *Introduction to Cell Biology*, Wadsworth Publishing, 1983.

Index

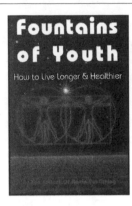

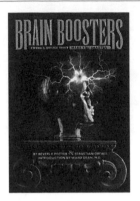

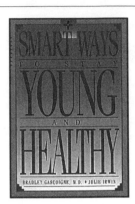

Fountains of Youth: How to Live Longer and Healthier Editors of Ronin Publishing 1996. Practical overview of nutrients, pharmaceuticals, and techniques that help you use recent gerontological breakthroughs to extend your life. How the aging process is reversed, antioxidants and megavitamins, herbal rejuvenators, and anti-aging pharmaceuticals.
Ronin   242 pp.
FOUYOU   **$14.95**

Brain Boosters: Foods and Drugs that Make You Smarter Potter and Orfali 1993. Fascinating look at foods and drugs that are reported to make the mind work better. For professionals, business people, seniors, people concerned with Alzheimer's and other neurological impairments, students, athletes, and party-goers who want to improve mental performance.
Ronin   257 pp.
BRABOO   **$14.95**

Smart Ways to Stay Young and Healthy Gascoigne and Irwin 1992. Sound advice on how to maintain physical and mental health. Brief chapters, each presenting one simple thing you can do for your well-being, youthfulness, and happiness. Tips include power naps, immunizing yourself, relaxation breathing exercises, stretching, and keeping your sex life happy.
Ronin   128 pp.
SMAWAY   **$7.95**

Finding a Path With a Heart: How to Go from Burnout to Bliss Beverly Potter 1995. Find direction and meaning in your work and life. Follow a path that is in tune with your values and your heart.
Ronin   356 pp.
FINPAT   **$14.95**

Beating Job Burnout: How to Transform Work Pressure into Productivity Beverly Potter 1993. Renew enthusiasm for work by developing personal power; recognize job burnout and overcome it.
Ronin   302 pp.
BEAJOB   **$14.95**

Chlorella: The Emerald Food Bewicke and Potter 19984. Amazing alchemist micro-algae supplies 19 essential amino acids, over 20 vitamins and minerals, and three times as much protein as beef.
Ronin   128 pp.
CHLORE   **$7.95**